Roberto Albani

Gastroesophageal reflux in children

Understanding and treating it

Dr Roberto Albani's practical guides

1

To my daughter Marta who suffered from gastroesophageal reflux before I knew how to help her.

CONTENTS

Introduction

You might be wondering why I decided to write a guide to gastroesophageal reflux when there are so many other conditions a paediatrician could choose to talk about. I've got some very sound reasons and I'll try to explain them to you.

Firstly, gastroesophageal reflux is one of the most common disorders in humans. Any book that helps people to spot the condition and treat it seems to me to be a very good thing for this reason alone. I have also had first hand experience of the trials and tribulations that trouble parents who happen to have a child with this problem. So it came natural to me to do what I could to help other parents avoiding the same mistakes I made in my initial ignorance.

In the 1970s, when my second daughter began to suffer from gastroesophageal reflux, hardly anyone knew about it, and I could do nothing to alleviate her suffering. However the experience served me well because I was able to make observations that I would otherwise have missed. These have helped me enormously in understanding and treating thousands of other children. Above all, they made me realize one fundamental thing: gastroesophageal reflux (GER), although almost never endangers a child's health and growth, can be an affliction that has very often a detrimental impact on the quality of life of the child and the whole family.

Paediatricians today distinguish between "physiological" reflux (GER, which affects 50-60 per cent of new-borns) and "gastroesophageal reflux disease" (GERD, which affects a small minority of children, but can have severe complications). Now, I think "Physiological reflux" (GER), is extremely underestimated and often dismissed as "nothing to worry about", in spite of the fact that can literally ruin the life of children and their families due to its intensity and persistence, with all the attendant emotional implications. And, having been able to follow my young patients into adulthood, I have realized how much this disorder continues to affect their lives even after early childhood. It has a big influence on their sleep and mood, significantly impacting their day-to-day lives.

This is why I believe it is always advisable to identify and treat the condition, even if the children who suffer from it are apparently well-nourished and in good health. And every day practice has taught me that it is almost never necessary to carry out invasive examinations such as pH monitoring, or esophagoscopy to diagnose the condition. The patient's history and symptoms, assessed by means of a simple questionnaire, help to establish a diagnosis with reasonable certainty in most cases.

Lastly, more than 40 years' experience with reflux has allowed me to develop a treatment method that usually works much better than those used by most of my colleagues. And, knowing very well what goes on in these families has allowed me to empathize with them, which is what many of them need most, having often felt misunderstood and neglected.

Roberto Albani

CHAPTER I

UNDERSTANDING REFLUX

What exactly is reflux?

In one of the photographs of my second daughter Marta, taken when she was three months old, she appears with a pale, sad little face and… a trickle of milk emerging from her mouth. This was the tell-tale sign of that period: **regurgitation** everywhere, on a multitude of bibs, on the shoulders of our clothes and on the carpet. And the smell of curdled milk, which is why we nicknamed Marta "little cheese". We marvelled at her ability to emit powerful **burps** even several hours after feeding, noises that made everyone laugh and earned her another nickname: the "navvy". She was also plagued by **hiccups** several times a day. She must have had them when she was still in her mother's belly, because the rhythmic jerking of her little body was clearly visible from outside.

All this, as well as colic, contortions and crying. Sometimes there was no way to comfort her. She seemed better only when held upright in our arms, with her body against our chests and her head on our shoulders. I remember that her face often looked as though she had given up hope and was resigned to feeling ill.

As time went on, the attacks we called **"colic"** did not abate but continued day and night. By the age of six months, Marta had stopped regurgitating all the time but started **vomiting** occasionally instead. She continued to get hiccups, although a little less often than before. She was still unsettled all the time, refusing to lie down and rest.

Rest? A luxury we never got to experience. Marta didn't sleep, or rather she woke up constantly and even in her sleep she twisted and turned in her cot as though possessed. She preferred to sleep on her tummy, with her little bottom stuck up in the air. Her tendency to burp long after she had eaten also stayed with her.

She began to walk unaided very early, at 10 months, and she began soon the habit of going around the house holding a bottle of apple juice or simple water and sucking continually on it. She wanted the bottle with her even when she was in bed, because at night she latched back onto it every time she woke up, as if she had an inextinguishable thirst. And at night, we continuously went to and fro between our room and hers, picking her up, comforting her, putting her dummy back in her mouth and waiting for her to drop back off. It was a torment for her and us. We were at the end of our tether, we'd had enough.

At that time, I was in New York doing my third year of postgraduate studies in paediatrics. I had a very good paediatric gastroenterologist on hand to ask for advice but even he couldn't offer me any help. "Marta is OK", he told me, "she looks healthy and is growing well. **There is nothing really wrong with her** …". Does this sound familiar to you?

A valve that doesn't work.

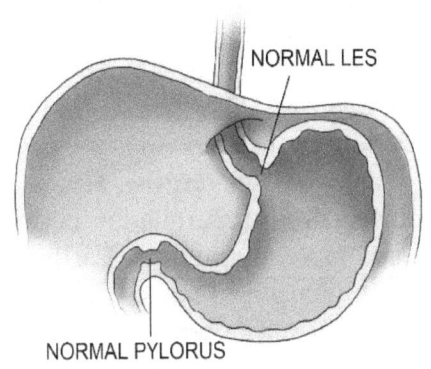

NORMAL LES

NORMAL PYLORUS

Figure 1

But what causes gastroesophageal reflux and why is it so frequent in babies? I have often fantasised that maybe it could be the consequence of an evolutionary deficiency in our species. I.e. maybe the valve between the oesophagus and the stomach, known as the *lower oesophageal sphincter (LES) (figure 1)* had probably not fully developed. It was as though we humans were originally ruminants and the structure of our oesophagus and stomach did not properly adapt when we turned into omnivores. When you see a newborn baby regurgitating continuously, it looks as though he or she is ruminating or chewing the cud. In fact, until a couple of decades ago the disorder was even known as *"merycism"* or "rumination syndrome".

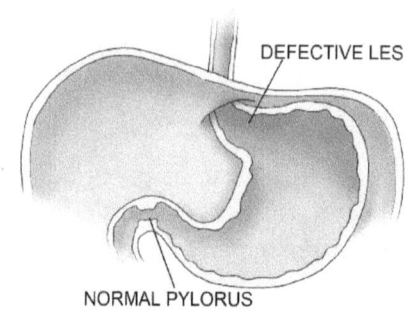

DEFECTIVE LES

NORMAL PYLORUS

Figure 1

Whether this is true or not, in children with reflux the LES often remains open or "patent" (figure 2), so that the stomach contents go back up towards the oesophagus for several hours after a meal. *Most of what goes up, though, is immediately re-swallowed.* Only a small portion reaches the mouth and is visibly regurgitated When this entire process is repeated day after day it inevitably leads to at least two consequences.

a. the oesophageal mucosa becomes increasingly irritated due to contact with gastric acid. This leads to *"oesophagitis"* and, besides causing obvious discomfort and pain, has several other consequences. It stimulates the phrenic nerve endings, causing *hiccupping.* The inflammation also affects the oesophageal muscles, occasionally causing *strong spasms and difficulty swallowing*. Oesophagitis also causes *nausea*, ultimately triggering attacks of *vomiting*. This differs from regurgitation because the food is expelled more abundantly and violently, in a jet. Lastly, the inflammation (exacerbated by the vomiting episodes) makes the tissues of the oesophagus more rigid so that the LES stays open for longer and the reflux gets worse. So the disorder enters into a *vicious cycle of worsening inflammation-increased reflux-exacerbated inflammation... and so on*.

b. the second consequence is that, particularly when lying down, *food that comes up can "go down the wrong way"*, in other words it might go down the trachea and in some rare cases even reach the smallest branches of the bronchi, with the attendant risk of *aspiration pneumonia*. Food inhalation can be severe enough to cause respiratory arrest, but this only happens very rarely.

Hiatus hernia

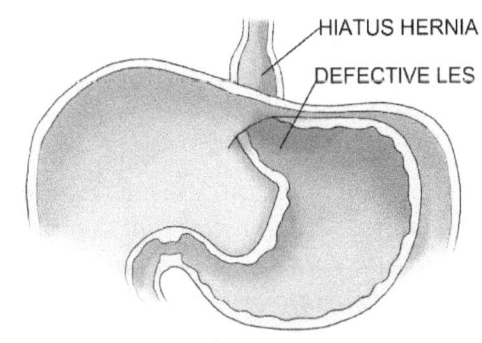

Figure 2

Reflux is very often associated with *hiatus hernia (figure 3)*. This happens when a small portion of the stomach slips from the abdomen into the thorax through a hole (hiatus) in the diaphragm muscle that in this case is much larger than it should be. In its normal size, this hole serves the purpose of letting the oesophagus through the diaphragm to connect with the stomach. The presence of the hernia allows the excessive opening of the LES and thus also reflux.

A hiatus hernia in children almost never requires surgery because in most cases it will disappear spontaneously as the child gets older.

In any case, most children with reflux display very clear symptoms of this disorder during the early months of life, also because they have a shorter oesophagus and the stomach contents do not have to travel much to reach the mouth.

Reflux, liquids, milk and sweet foods

It goes without saying that *the presence of moderate quantities of liquids in the stomach is one of the factors promoting reflux,* since liquids pass much more easily than solids through the patent LES. This is one of the reasons why reflux is particularly active in newborns, who feed exclusively on milk. This situation does not change at the beginning of weaning, because even in this phase babies *still feed mainly on milk.*

Cow's milk-based infant formulas make reflux worse

Babies who are exclusively breast-fed, even if they regurgitate frequently, usually begin to suffer from reflux later than the ones who are fed formula. These babies, in fact, begin to vomit and become unsettled soon after they start formula feedings. Many of my colleagues mistakenly interpret this as a sign that reflux is due to *intolerance to the protein in milk*. I think another explanation is much more likely. *When digesting the protein in cow's milk formula, the stomach needs to produce definitely more acidity than that required to digest breast milk*. Closer inspection reveals that regurgitation following breast milk is fluid, watery and inoffensive smelling, while regurgitation after formula feeding contains bigger curds and emits a strong acid smell. *I am sure that the rapid worsening of symptoms in children fed on formula milk is almost always due to this mechanism rather than to a supposed "intolerance"*.

Sweet foods make reflux worse

Experience has also taught me that *sweet foods*, including fruit-based baby foods, accentuate gastric acidity and therefore worsen reflux or make it flare up when latent.

Many children continue to suffer from reflux until adulthood

When the baby is about six months old, the reflux usually changes. This may be because the oesophagus lengthens and the stomach settles better into the abdomen as the baby grows rapidly, or it could be because the diet becomes more solid as weaning starts. From the moment children begin to stand and walk, they usually keep down food more and more effectively due to their more upright position. This means that the stomach contents are less likely to rise back up into the oesophagus and reach the mouth as easily as during the first few months. *In other words, the situation becomes more similar to typical adult reflux: regurgitation takes still place but is less frequent and less visible*.

In other words, despite the apparent improvement, very often the acid reflux continues to occur and cause problems even once the child is over one year old.

Many children with reflux continue to bring up acid, particularly when lying down. A significant proportion of them ultimately continue to suffer from reflux until they are adults, experiencing flare-ups interspersed with periods of well-being.

It is estimated that in the USA, no fewer than 10 million adults, i.e. approximately *3 per cent of the population* complain of heartburn *on a daily basis,*. This does not include people who suffer from the same symptoms sporadically or have difficulty in swallowing, sleep disturbances, frequent burping, nausea in the morning and so on. All these signs usually indicate a milder form of the condition and affect a much greater proportion of the population, which can be as much as *15 to 20 per cent*. So, what does this mean?

It means that, *based on the fact that approximately 50 per cent of newborns show clear symptoms of reflux, half of these go on to suffer from the same symptoms into adulthood, albeit sporadically and more subtly.*

What external factors promote reflux?

Several disorders can accentuate reflux, with a direct or indirect effect on its mechanisms.

a. *Respiratory tract infection with coughing* is one of the most common. Coughing involves abrupt contractions of the diaphragm, which presses on the stomach and pushes its contents up toward the oesophagus, ultimately causing vomiting. This mechanism often causes a recurrence of reflux in children who have apparently recovered from the disorder, because it sets the vicious cycle of vomiting-oesophagitis-reflux-more vomiting in motion again.

b. A similar mechanism may be triggered if the child contracts *gastroenteritis*, which always begins with repeated episodes of vomiting.

c. A *diet rich in* sweet foods, or *sweetened drinks clearly promotes reflux*.

d. *"Is reflux hereditary?"* is one of the most common questions asked by the parents of young reflux sufferers My answer is yes, simply because the shape and function of the LES valve are genetic traits, like the shape of the nose or ears. So it is reasonable to expect that, *if one of the parents suffers from a particularly intense form of reflux, at least some of their children will have the same problem*.

CHAPTER II

REFLUX DURING THE FIRST SIX MONTHS

The most common symptoms

Reflux is unlikely to show clear signs of its presence during the first days of life because, even if the preconditions are present, *it takes some time for oesophagitis to develop*.

Regurgitation

At birth, therefore, the first sign is simply a tendency to *regurgitate frequently*, but almost without any discomfort or suffering. What is the difference between "regurgitating frequently" and the sporadic spitting up typical of almost all normal newborns? It means *regurgitating more often and more abundantly, almost after each feed.*

If babies are breast-fed, for the reasons explained above, those with frequent regurgitation may not show signs of discomfort even for the first two or three months. By contrast, babies *fed on formula* begin to show significant signs of suffering almost immediately.

Painful attacks

In any case, sooner or later, all of them become unsettled and then experience painful attacks, causing them to cry intermittently for hours. These attacks are usually mistakenly *called "colic".*

As time passes, the baby will *regurgitate* more and more often and even several hours following a feed, perhaps when you are just getting ready to give the next feed.

Vomiting

Sometimes the baby will have episodes of *projectile vomiting*. In more acute cases, this can simulate a different disorder that is much rarer than reflux, known as *hypertrophic pyloric stenosis* (I will explain the different later).

Hiccupping

From the outset, the baby suffers from *persistent hiccupping* after nearly every feed. This is one of the most characteristic signs of oesophagitis. It is the very inflammation of the oesophagus that stimulates the phrenic nerve endings, thus triggering the rhythmic contraction of the diaphragm.

Most children who suffer from reflux actually give advance warning of their disorder by *hiccupping before birth* when they are still in their mother's belly.

Wind, burping and difficulty in feeding

The baby *burps* frequently, often hours after a meal, due to the large quantity of air swallowed in the intervals between feeds as he or she continually gulps back the milk that comes up. Perhaps due to the sensation of being bloated by all this air or due to swallowing difficulties caused by the oesophagitis, the baby *is very unsettled while feeding.* So feeds often turn into battles with the breast (or bottle). The baby latches on for a few minutes, then suddenly stiffens, kicks, breaks away and cries in evident frustration. Despite wanting to feed quickly, he or she is unable to and ultimately gives up the struggle after a few minutes of this performance. Then the baby begins to protest hungrily after half an hour to an hour and latches back on to finish feeding. This can go on and on in a continuous loop, reducing the mother to the brink of exhaustion because she has no time at all to rest.

None of this is life-threatening, of course, but let's try to put ourselves in the shoes of the poor baby and mother. All this unpleasantness does not give them much to be cheerful about. Since I personally experienced this problem with my own daughter, I have noticed that the eyes of these babies express what you would expect in their situation: pain, irritation and resignation.

The baby grows normally

Despite this unenviable situation, apart from the odd rare case, children with reflux manage to get enough nutrition and grow normally. This means that their suffering (and that of their family) is often unfairly overlooked and paediatricians will dismiss concerns with comments such as: *"Don't go looking for problems. Your baby is growing nicely, there's nothing wrong!"* Along the same lines, most of my gastroenterologist colleagues only classify reflux as *GERD, "GastroEsophageal Reflux Disease"* (and therefore worthy of attention and treatment) if it is accompanied by complications such as stunted growth, aspiration pneumonia, severe oesophagitis etc. Therefore, according to this definition, only a very small percentage of children with the painful disorder I see every day would deserve attention.

The baby wants to be held all the time

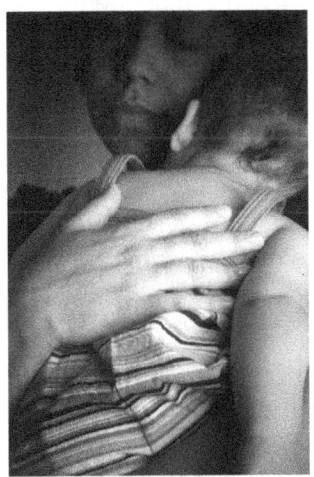 When I see a child with reflux for the first time, the scene that unfolds before me is always the same, with a few minor variations. One of the parents talks to me while the other holds the baby upright with its head resting on his or her shoulder and paces around the room. If he/she sits down and tries to place the baby in a more horizontal position, the baby immediately begins to squirm and cry angrily. I no longer Now, I very well know that this behaviour goes on throughout the day at home and believe that it is one of the toughest consequences of gastroesophageal reflux. Parents naturally do not want to leave the baby crying inconsolably. This is totally understandable but leads inevitably to habits that will be very difficult to break even once the reflux is finally cured or has cleared up spontaneously.

Temperament, anxious parents and reflux

When you observe children who regurgitate, you will often notice that some of them appear happy and smiling, while others seem to suffer more even though they show significantly fewer signs of reflux. This shows that the degree of suffering is also very dependent on the *tolerance threshold of each individual child*. In particular, I think that children *with a more demanding and sensitive temperament* perceive and manifest the discomforts associated with reflux to a greater extent.

Conversely, it is also clear that *very anxious parents* may over-estimate their child's discomfort.

Can the child choke due to regurgitation and vomiting? Can it cause coughing and respiratory infections?

Over several decades of experience with many young reflux patients, I have only seen a severe chocking episode once, when a five-month-old baby suffered a sudden, massive inhalation of vomit and a respiratory arrest, which ultimately caused extensive brain damage. I should point out, however, that this child had a very serious case of reflux that had not been properly treated. In other words, such an occurrence is extremely unlikely and appropriate treatment reduces this risk to zero in any case. Nevertheless, it is quite common for minute amounts of regurgitated milk or food to come into contact with the larynx. This explains why, particularly when in a horizontal position, the child experiences the following:

- *sudden, sporadic coughing spells.*
- during the years of nursery school, when he/she continually catches respiratory viruses, will develop more easily than others *laryngitis, bronchitis and bronchiolitis.*
- possible episodes of *bronchial asthma.*

But appropriate treatment for reflux will also minimize the incidence of these respiratory complications.

Vagal hyperstimulation with near-fainting spells.

Shortly after I began my practice, the mother of Mirco, a four month old baby with reflux, called me in great alarm. "My baby has passed out, he's stopped reacting!" she wailed down the phone. I tried to explain what was happening, but she was too upset. I asked her to bring her baby to see me straight away. She told me that Mirco had suddenly become very pale and apparently collapsed, without completely losing consciousness. She admitted that she had deliberately stopped her baby's reflux treatment a week before because he seemed well. I didn't discover anything of significance during my examination and was unable to explain the event at that stage. I still advised the mother to resume treatment, because it seemed likely that the episode had something to do with the reflux. Since then, I have often received similar phone calls and have also discovered that the phenomenon is definitely linked to oesophagitis. Intense irritation of the mucosa can cause these strange episodes through stimulation of the vagus nerve endings (the vagus is another nerve associated with the oesophagus). Symptoms include *a feeling of extreme weakness, intense pallor and slowing of the heart rate to the point that the child appears to be unconscious*. However, all this happens only sporadically and only to children with more intense forms of oesophagitis. The phenomenon is not serious in its own right, but parents are understandably scared because they mistake it for fainting and are afraid that their child is on the brink of expiring before their eyes.

What does constipation have to do with reflux?

Constipation became my daughter Marta's main problem when she was about four months old, coinciding with the time she started taking supplements of formula milk. As if the regurgitation, hiccups and "colic" weren't enough, the poor little thing had to cope with this new difficulty as well. The longer she went without moving her bowels, the harder her stools became and the more she instinctively held it in to avoid the pain of evacuation. At that time, I had no way of knowing what many years of experience subsequently taught me, i.e. that constipation is linked to reflux. You may well ask what link there can possibly be between the function of the LES at the entrance to the digestive system and that of the anal sphincter at the other end. I've asked myself the same thing and never found an answer with any scientific basis. I eventually decided that it could be the consequence of nervous tension triggered by the oesophagitis, which makes it difficult for the baby to relax and open the anal sphincter to let the stool out. Whatever the reason, constipation often becomes an additional cause of distress for these children.

Reflux without any reflux.

Many children show all the signs of reflux without exhibiting its more obvious symptoms. Above all, they do not display frequent regurgitation, which is a classic sign, allowing easy diagnosis. Even without regurgitation, a child with reflux will display one of the following: *frequent hiccups, "colic" and/or sporadic episodes of projectile vomiting*.

23

However, with all the chat about reflux on the Internet, I quite often see children whose parents are "certain" that they have reflux just because they cry frequently, though I often find out they are suffering from other problems.

Can reflux stop children from eating enough?

One of the main concerns expressed by the mothers who come to me is that reflux is preventing their child from eating enough.

It is actually rare for a child to end up not eating enough simply due to reflux. Only if he/she suffers from a particularly severe form of GERD, like the one that follows surgery for oesophageal atresia, i.e. congenital obstruction of part of the oesophagus.

What is the difference between reflux and pyloric stenosis?

Hypertrophic pyloric stenosis (figure 4), is a serious disease and much

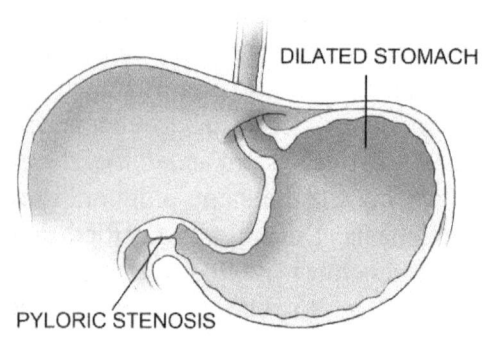

rarer than reflux. It is a progressive narrowing of the pyloric sphyncter, at the point where the stomach joins the gut. Statistics tell us that approximately one in every 500 newborns has it. The disorder is much rarer in baby girls (only approximately 1/2000 of whom get it) than baby boys.

Day after day, gradual obstruction of the pylorus increasingly prevents normal stomach emptying, causing uncontainable *projectile vomiting*, when *the child expels the entire stomach contents in a jet that can reach up to one and a half metres.* In such cases, reflux treatments can bring about a slight improvement for a day or two. But as time goes on, the vomiting gets worse, eventually causing *dehydration and malnutrition.*

DILATED STOMACH

PYLORIC STENOSIS

Figure 4

24

Because the progress of symptoms is so much more dramatic than in cases of reflux, this disorder can easily be identified without further investigation. In this case, ultrasound diagnosis is decisive, because it clearly shows the obstructed pylorus and the enlarged muscle surrounding it. Hypertrophic pyloric stenosis can only be resolved by simple surgery.

REFLUX DURING THE FIRST SIX MONTHS

In my experience, we can easily diagnose gastroesophageal reflux in babies by observing its symptoms, as one does for the common cold. If babies regurgitate frequently (after each feed), always have hiccups, vomit

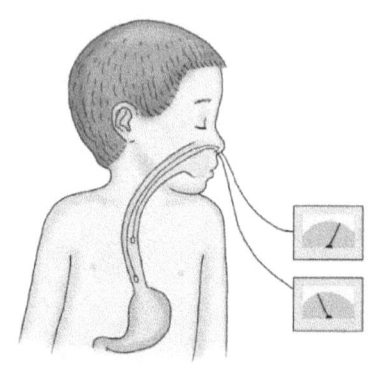

from time to time, have "colic" and are unsettled when feeding, there is no doubt that they are suffering from reflux IF ALL THESE SYMPTOMS OCCUR TOGETHER. However, many of my colleagues believe it necessary to carry out an instrumental examination in any case, such as an ultrasound scan or pH test (figure 5).

I personally think that these tests are hardly ever essential and not even always reliable. Reflux *varies greatly from moment to moment* and its actual

Figure 5

relevance may not be fully apparent during a particular tests. *Actually, when carrying out a pH tests, the presence of a probe in the oesophagus may be even a confounding factor. In fact, it gives the baby an intense feeling of a foreign body,* which may trigger retching, and/or vomiting and prevent the child from feeding normally, affecting the outcome one way or another. For these reasons, I rely much more on parents' observations. Following the example of other academics I drew up a questionnaire that can be used to make the diagnosis and monitor the progress of reflux without resorting to expensive and/or invasive tests.

My questionnaire allocates a certain score to each symptom, based on its presence and intensity. If the overall score obtained exceeds the specified maximum level of normality, we can conclude that the child has reflux. In this case, specialist referral is needed to confirm the diagnosis and begin treatment.

WARNING. *Because many of the symptoms you will find listed in the following questionnaire are generic, you must identify at least one of the symptoms specific to the disorder before reaching conclusions on reflux in your child. These symptoms are indicated in bold and under-lined:*

QUESTIONNAIRE FOR THE FIRST SIX MONTHS

1. Does your child experience **frequent regurgitation, sometimes up to several hours after feeding**? (Regurgitation means acid milk emerging from the mouth without any effort, not in a jet)
   2 to 5 times per day.............3 points
   5 or more times..................5 points

2. Does your child seem to re-swallow **the acid, as though chewing the cud?**
   2 to 5 times per day............2 points
   5 to 10 times...................5 points

3. Has **hiccups** more than once a day?
   1 to 3 times a day...........3 points
   4 or more....................5 points

4. Burps frequently, sometimes several hours after feeding?
   2 to 4 times per day...........2 points
   5 or more.....................5 points

5. Has **recurrent episodes of projectile vomiting**?
   1 per week...................3 points
   2 or more....................5 points

6. Is constantly unsettled ("can't keep still") when waking and asleep?
   no......0 points   yes.........2 points

7. Has "**"colic""**, bouts of crying due to pain that the paediatrician cannot explain otherwise?
   from time to time.........1 point
   1 or more per day..........5 points

8. Often "difficult" to feed, disturbed by frequent stiffening and back-arching, crying and detaching from the breast (or bottle) and breaking off despite being evidently hungry?
   Once daily...................2 points
   More than once..............3 points

9. Tends to hold his or her neck cocked to one side, which can give the impression of a muscular or neurological problem?
   sometimes....................2 points
   usually.........................4 points

10. Sleeps in a disturbed and unsettled manner and wakes up constantly. Cannot rest for more than two or three hours at a time?
    No.....0 points   yes......4 points

If you score **more than 10** on the questionnaire, your child probably has gastro-esophageal reflux. Don't forget: **to suspect reflux at least one of the specific signs highlighted in bold and underlined must be present under all circumstances.**

TREATING REFLUX DURING THE FIRST SIX MONTHS

Postural therapy

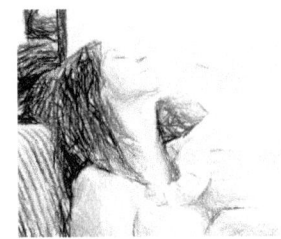

All parents soon realize that babies with reflux feel better when they are held as upright as possible, because this greatly reduces the amount of acid that comes back up from the stomach and allows the stomach to empty down toward the intestine.

The problem is that such babies usually end up being held by their parents from dawn to dusk, apart from a few short intervals when they manage to sleep lying down. So this habit can easily become a vice that is very difficult to break at a later stage, even once the reflux has improved considerably.

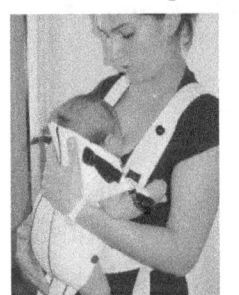

For this reason, I always advise parents to equip themselves with items that they can use to keep their babies in a comfortable position without having to hold them all the time.

For example, one basic rule that will significantly help reduce the acid reflux to the oesophagus and empty the stomach more effectively, is to resort to the "baby wearing", using a **sling** or a **baby carrier** as soon as possible, from the first days of life. This will not harm his/her back or hips in the least, particularly with the ergonomic baby carriers on sale today. Adults caring for babies can carry them around in this way throughout the day, just as African women have done for centuries. Because less acid comes up from the stomach using this method, the oesophagus becomes progressively less inflamed and there is less

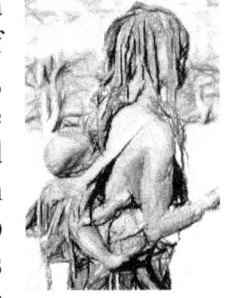

likelihood of having to use drugs to counteract the stomach acid.

Because, this very effective anti-reflux method cannot be used at night for obvious reasons, for more than 10 years I have been developing a device that will hold the child in the same position without having to be held by a person. This will be available a few months after this edition of my book is issued.

How to manage feeds

Breast-feeding only

What happens if the mother feeds her baby exclusively on breastmilk, as everyone would in an ideal world? Simple: a baby with reflux will get a head's start. During digestion, breast milk triggers less acid secretion, meaning that regurgitation is less irritating to the oesophagus than that following formula milk. Symptoms are therefore milder and appear at a later stage.

For this reason, mothers of children with reflux should always be encouraged to continue with breast-feeding for as long as possible.

Thickening top-up feeds does not improve the situation

I am often asked whether it is useful to thicken any top-up feeds of formula milk. *I reply that this does not work and can even be counterproductive, so it is better to top up with liquid milk.*

Thickened formula milk

If you are forced to stop breastfeeding and use only formula milk, then it is better to use a thickened form of it, which will stay better and longer in the stomach due to gravity. You could try an *anti-reflux or AR formula*, which contains carob flour and other thickeners and usually does the job effectively. Or you can thicken liquid infant formula yourself at home to achieve comparable results much more cheaply. In which case I advise the following preparation method:

Ingredients:
1. Powder or liquid infant formula
2. **Rice flour or maize starch (cornflour) and tapioca starch**. Choose the option that the child seems to like the most, or even rotate them to break the monotony. Make sure you choose an unsweetened flour.

If you use **powdered milk**, make up the mixture by adding one scoop of powder and one scoop of flour for each 30 cc of water (or 60, if the milk instructions are for this quantity). Follow these proportions whatever the final overall quantity. I advise using a stick blender to obtain a smooth mixture.

If you use **liquid formula**, always add one scoop of flour (use a powder formula scoop) for each 30 cc (or grams) of formula, then blend.

Experiment for a while with different flour quantities *in order to make a gel of yoghurt -like consistency*.

This thickened milk obviously cannot pass through the holes of a normal teat, so it must be replaced by one with a *star or Y-cut teat*, of the type usually adopted to give babies their first solid meal.

Soy milk?

I have noticed that many babies *improve faster if they drink soy or rice milk, particularly at the beginning of treatment*. This is not because they are allergic or intolerant to cow's milk (which forms the basis of usual infant formulas), but because soy or rice milk becomes less acid when digested. If the baby seems to respond positively to this type of milk, I advise continuing to give it for at least a few weeks, then try a cow's milk-based formula when the reflux symptoms are well under control.

How much milk do I prepare?

Simple: feed your baby until he or she is full, remembering that *the reflux does not depend on how much milk the baby takes*.

Thickened milk, questions and objections:

1. "Isn't it too much for a newborn to take a feed that is already so thick and so full of rice/corn and tapioca starch?"
2. "Aren't there too many carbohydrates and calories in this baby food? Won't it cause obesity?"

My answer is that 40 years of experience have shown me that children following this regime show a distinct improvement in their reflux, digest food well and grow normally without getting fat.

Will my baby need to drink more?

The water contained in the milk, even when thickened, is usually perfectly sufficient to meet the child's needs under normal temperature conditions. If it is very hot and the baby is evidently thirsty (i.e. drinks the water greedily), small sips are the best rule. Give 5-10 ml of water at a time, many times a day if necessary. In this way, the baby will drink all the water needed without triggering an increase in reflux.

Will weaning improve the symptoms? And when should I start?

Many parents ask if it is appropriate to introduce solid food more quickly in the belief that this might bring about an instant improvement in the reflux. I inevitably reply that their expectations are groundless and that it is not at all a good idea to hasten weaning.

If the mother is feeding her baby exclusively on breastmilk, *introducing a single solid meal usually makes the situation worse. You have to consider in fact, that the milk of the previous feeding remains in the stomach for several hours and therefore mixes with the oncoming solid food and dilutes it. Because solid food triggers more acid secretion, the result is that acid reflux increases and causes its well-known consequences.*

So I always recommend feeding exclusively on breast milk until the sixth month. This is in any case what experts recommend, even for children who do not have any problems, and there are plenty of good reasons for this.

If the child is taking thickened formula milk, early weaning is perfectly welcome, as the baby is already eating solid food.

How to start weaning

For children with reflux *I definitely advise against introducing fruit and above all jarred fruit,* which tends to worsen symptoms due to its sugar content. Instead I start by directly introducing savoury baby food, in other words a blend of vegetables, creamed cereals, blended or freeze-dried meat, according to the baby's tastes and appetite. From then on, weaning a baby with reflux is no different from weaning any other baby.

What about medicines?

It is important to remember that the measures I have described so far, though essential to reach a good result, do not usually by themselves resolve the problem but amount to 50 per cent of the solution. Therefore, if the baby with reflux shows signs of considerable discomfort, I personally consider that, in spite of the fact that we are dealing with GER and not GERD, the suffering is such that it deserves almost always treatment with medicines.

Two types of drugs work well for this purpose. Firstly, drugs that inhibit acid secretion by the stomach mucosa (**antisecretory drugs**) and secondly drugs that neutralize the acid once it has been produced (**antacids**).

Antisecretory drugs

The most effective and most commonly used agents of this type are **proton pump inhibitors**, which can limit acidity for most of the day following a single dose. These include omeprazole, lansoprazole, esomeprazole, pantoprazole and rabeprazole sodium.

Other drugs are sold for a similar purpose (cimetidine and ranitidine) but I believe them to be considerably less effective than the ones mentioned above, and they come with at least as many possible side effects.

Antacids

The most effective antacids I have come across in my long years of experience are those based on aluminium and magnesium hydroxide, available in different forms and brands in different countries (such as Maalox, Riopan, Gelusil etc.). The right dose of each of these can neutralize acid produced by the stomach for several hours. This means that regurgitation will not irritate the oesophageal mucosa during this time interval. These antacids have no demonstrable harmful effects and can be used without fear.

How can I decide which of these drugs to give and in what doses?

First try antacids alone

My own rule of thumb is as follows:

If I think the reflux is mild, *I try giving antacids alone*, choosing one based on the child's personal taste. Because the treatment will be long-term, it is important for the child to like the taste of the medicine.

I prescribe a dose of at least 3 ml (increased up to 5 ml), to be administered up to six or seven times daily, immediately before each feed. Remember: *immediately before the feed and not afterwards*, because babies are more likely to take the medicine willingly when they are hungry. They are also more likely to keep it down and not vomit it, as often happens if they take it after feeding. However, *you can choose to give the drug after feeding, or during breaks in feeding, according to what seems to suit your baby best*.

Is the aluminium in the antacids harmful?

Why do some of my colleagues advise against taking aluminium-based antacids, saying that this element can accumulate in the bloodstream and become toxic to the brain?

Let's take a look at the facts. This is what experts have written on the absorption and toxicity of drugs containing aluminium hydroxide:

*During the action of aluminium and magnesium hydroxide (i.e. Maalox, Gelusil, Riopan) on stomach acid, small quantities of magnesium and aluminium are released. These are converted during their passage through the gut to **relatively insoluble phosphates and eliminated in this form in the faeces. The very small portion of aluminium absorbed (1 per cent), is quickly eliminated in the urine.***

***Only subjects with severely impaired kidney function (such as people on dialysis) might accumulate aluminium**.*

Personally, I would add that, *even though drugs such as Maalox, Gelusil or Riopan have been used extensively for decades, not one case of aluminium toxicity due to these drugs has been described in the medical literature* (except, as stated previously, in people with severe kidney impairment).

34

When should antisecretory drugs be added.

When your child has very severe symptoms (the questionnaire score significantly exceeds 16) and/or does not seem any better after a few days of treatment with antacids alone, I would advise *adding an antisecretory agent* without stopping the antacids.

I almost always prescribe *lansoprazole at a dose of 7 to 15 mg*, to be given in the morning before breakfast. Orally soluble tablets are available. These are made up of granules that can be diluted in a few cc of water and given with a teaspoon or syringe.

I recommend continuing the antacids indefinitely but try to taper off antisecretory agents gradually after several weeks of administration. If the symptoms flare up again, I re-introduce the antisecretory agents for as long as seems necessary, periodically attempting to stop giving them.

How long does it take for the child to get better after starting treatment?

The benefits are usually already evident after the first 24 hours of treatment and reach a maximum within one week. *Be warned, however, when children begin to take thickened milk at home, they may experience a few episodes of projectile vomiting during the first two or three days*, giving the impression that the condition may even have worsened. In this case, just carry on without making any changes and the problem will clear up within a few days.

In any case, I always advise parents not to become alarmed if the child experiences a sudden return of symptoms for one or two days despite being much better generally, because *reflux is subject to spontaneous fluctuations* and may have such surprises in store. Just carry on with the treatment, possibly adding an extra dose of antacid at the worse times to overcome these temporary attacks.

How to treat constipation in reflux cases.

As I have already explained, constipation is a very common symptom in children with reflux and *usually appears when using formula milk or when a breast-fed baby starts to be weaned*. The problem can usually be resolved by simply treating the reflux properly using the methods described above.

Despite such treatment, some children continue to have difficulty eliminating somewhat hard stools and experience evident discomfort. To prevent babies from being drawn into a vicious cycle that could mean they do not pass any stools for days on end, I would act as soon as possible to help. Fortunately, nowadays it is possible to obtain absolutely harmless substances that can soften the stools without causing side effects or addiction. I personally choose either *lactulose or macrogol*. These substances can be found in a variety of powders or syrups. They can be added to the milk in the proportion of one teaspoonful per feed and this will make the stools much softer within a few days. Then I recommend increasing or decreasing the dose over the next week according to the response to find the right quantity. Keep giving the medicine for at least a couple of months to stabilize the outcome. After you stop giving the product, I recommend starting it again whenever the constipation recurs, safe in the knowledge that these substances are not proper drugs. Remember that they do not have significant side effects and will not cause addiction.

What should I do if a cough makes the reflux worse?

In this situation, I normally advise a couple of extra doses of antacid per day, administered in the intervals between feeds, and implementing postural therapy as much possible in a sling or baby carrier by day. I hope to be able to offer a nighttime solution shortly, as already mentioned.

What happens when viral gastroenteritis makes the reflux worse?

This situation is very risky, because when children with reflux contract gastroenteritis they can easily fall into a vicious cycle of vomiting-more oesophagitis-more vomiting.

If babies cannot take more fluids, they are even more at risk of the dehydration that is already possible with this type of infection. For this reason, I always advise taking immediate action when a baby with reflux begins to display symptoms of gastroenteritis. How?

36

a. *If the baby vomits repeatedly, it is advisable to starve completely of solids and liquids* for up to half a day, even if the baby seems hungry and thirsty. Do this until the baby stops suffering from bouts of spontaneous vomiting, i.e. vomiting not caused by ingesting anything.

b. *To prevent the oesophagitis getting worse, it is advisable to administer small quantities of antacid immediately*, (1-2 ml) every half-hour throughout the first day of illness, even if the baby continues to vomit.

c. *After a couple of hours, it is a good idea to supplement this treatment by beginning to offer teaspoonfuls of a salt solution for rehydration but don't insist if he or she doesn't seem to like it.*

d. *Breast-fed babies can breastfeed again once they have not vomited for at least a couple of hours. However, if they take formula milk, it is best to wait for a day before beginning to feed again. And it is better to feed with a lactose-free milk such as soy formula and re-introduce the usual milk on the following day.*

If the child vomits up everything eaten and drunk for more than 24 hours despite all these measures, they must be taken to the emergency room of a paediatric hospital.

What should I do if my child continues to cry despite all the treatment?

Remember that reflux symptoms are more pronounced in more sensitive children with a low pain tolerance threshold. I personally have the impression that this is why many children with reflux *complain a lot, even if they are being effectively treated.*

Or, even if the treatment is effective, many children get *so used to being picked up that they carry on crying just because they want to be held all the time. This is clear when* they immediately calm down and might even reward you with a smile as soon as they have what they want.

Other children might have different reasons for their discomfort. For example, many children *do not like being covered up too much and* scream in desperation when they are wearing too many layers. As soon as I begin to undress them, they seem to relax more and more, almost heaving a sigh of relief and giving me a beaming smile when they are finally naked.

From the age of six-seven months, the discomfort could also be caused by teething. This is sometimes easily identifiable but sometimes not.

So, when a child with reflux continues to cry despite being given the most effective treatments, I offer the following guidelines, which usually solve at least part of the problem:

1. *Avoid holding your child all the time*. After feeding, cleaning, dressing etc. and enjoying a few cuddles, you should go back to what you were doing before, despite any protests. If you can keep your cool, your baby might get the message and gradually get used to being a little more self-sufficient.

2. *Make sure to avoid covering him/her with too much clothing, as this in itself can cause discomfort and agitation.*

Pointless and/or damaging treatments

Before they get to see a specialist, children with reflux have often begun to take treatments prescribed by their general practitioner. Many of these are appropriate and effective. However, in just as many cases the child will have been prescribed absolutely inappropriate diets and drugs that are often counterproductive.

Diets for which there is no good evidence

I can only try to hammer home the point that *there is no evidence that reflux is usually caused by a food intolerance or allergy.* So I cannot justify the practice followed by many of my colleagues of using special formulas, including very expensive hydrolysed formulas. Countless children have come to me for treatment after switching milk several times without any benefit, and then improved in a few days after returning to a diet of thickened normal milk and the treatments I have described above. Therefore, unless there is incontrovertible evidence that the child has an allergy to milk proteins (i.e. symptoms such as vomiting, diarrhoea and breaking out in a skin rash over the entire body immediately after feeding) I think it is entirely unjustifiable to change to a special milk. *The only good reason for avoiding a cow's milk-based formula is, as I have already explained, the greater acidity that this causes during digestion. This is the only reason why I sometimes temporarily switch to a soy or rice-based formula when I begin treatment for reflux.*

Should breast-feeding mothers follow a special diet?

I think the advice often given to breast-feeding mothers to follow a diet free of cow's milk and dairy products is an absolute travesty. Many have adopted this measure based on outdated research showing that breast milk contains infinitesimal traces of ingested protein and it is clinically pointless as well as potentially harmful to the mother. This is another situation where I can describe countless cases where, having established that the measure was pointless, I told the mothers they did not need to bother following the diet and cleared up the child's reflux using the treatments described above.

Drugs that are of little use

Some medicines are habitually used instead of the antacids I mentioned. These products are usually based on alginates, i.e. substances that supposedly create a gelatinous plug in the LES when they come into contact with gastric acid. A gel does form, but it is not sufficiently effective to alleviate the symptoms, at least in the majority of children I have treated. For this reason, I don't usually resort to them at all. If I do use them, I give them in conjunction with antacids to enhance their effect.

TREATMENT FAQS

Can antacid cause diarrhoea?

Yes, magnesium hydroxide and some excipients in the antacids can cause a few more liquid stools than usual, up to five or six a day. However, this effect causes neither dehydration nor loss of nutrients. Quite the contrary, it helps the baby move its bowels more easily and resolves the problem of constipation typical of many reflux babies. It also makes it easy to get rid of wind, which is very uncomfortable for reflux babies, as we have seen. You can therefore relax and ignore this effect unless the baby moves its bowels more than six times per day.

What do I do if my baby gets worse despite being treated?

It's advisable to add one or two doses of antacids, even between feeds, for a few days. Go back to the usual dosage as soon as the baby is better.

What do I do if my baby doesn't like the taste of the antacid?

In this case, don't give up and abandon the treatment, otherwise the symptoms will come back as before. But it's also pointless to carry on with the same product, hoping that your baby will accept it eventually. It's best to try another medicine. For example, if your baby just doesn't like Maalox, you could try with Maalox plus, Riopan or Gadral, which are generally more palatable. In the end you'll always be able to find a product that your baby will take more willingly.

What do I do if my baby won't eat thickened milk?

First of all, check that the cut in the teat is big enough to allow your baby to suck out the thickened milk without any problems. The next step is to check that you haven't thickened the milk too much. It should have a yoghurt-like consistency. Try with another type of flour, e.g. corn and tapioca flour, or carob flour or alternatively perhaps both mixed together. To give your baby time to adapt to the new taste, don't worry too much if he or she eats a little less for a few days

Can I thicken breast milk?

Using a breast pump for months in order to thicken breast milk with flour is a considerable sacrifice, but some of my patients' mothers have done it and found this to be an acceptable solution. So why not have a go at this option before you give up trying to feed your baby with your own breast milk?

Can I allow my baby to sleep on his stomach, which is what he prefers?
I remember that when my second daughter was born in New York, the nurses immediately placed her on her stomach. This was common practice at the time in the USA because observations had shown that newborns cried less and slept better in that position. Unfortunately, research conducted in various European countries at the start of the 1990s showed a clear link between the "prone" position and cot death. Nowadays, we paediatricians must advise against placing babies on their stomachs until they are six months old and able to roll over to find their most comfortable position.

How will I know when my child is better? What tests should I do?
Many parents make an independent decision to stop treatment when they see that their baby is no longer displaying evident signs of reflux. I can understand their impatience, but unfortunately experience tells me that reflux almost never clears up spontaneously within the first six months. In any case, I believe it is a good idea to use the above questionnaire to find out the status of the disorder. No instrumental tests, including ultrasounds or invasive pH testing can establish the status of the disorder better than close observation by parents and completion of the questionnaire.

CHAPTER III

REFLUX FROM SIX MONTHS TO ONE YEAR

Children regurgitate less but vomit occasionally. They still hiccup.

After the beginning of weaning, between five and six months of age, reflux babies usually regurgitate less and find it so much easier to feed that they might seem "cured". At least this is what many parents conclude and therefore take a unilateral decision to stop treatment. Another reason is that they are concerned about giving their child medicines for such long periods, despite my reassurances that they are basically harmless.

Regurgitation, vomiting and hiccups.

They usually have to think again, though, if the child continues to suffer despite being apparently cured. Some lingering *regurgitation* and the occasional episode of *vomiting*, together with annoying *hiccupping* indicate the condition is still present.

Burping

Children also give an impression of *always having food sitting heavily on their stomachs* and struggling to digest it. They will often *burp several hours after a meal*.

Food cut into small pieces causes bouts of vomiting

As the months go by, reflux babies usually *will not accept food cut up into small pieces as other babies do.* If the food contains bits, however small, they will tend to cause bouts retching and vomiting. The explanation is that even though the oesophagitis may be mild, it makes the oesophagus more sensitive and causes it to go into spasm when swallowing solid food fragments. In other words, a mild form of *dysphagia* occurs.

Noisy swallowing

For the same reason, when swallowing, the child sometimes produces *a gurgling noise*, as though the food is going down with difficulty, between spasms and attacks of wind.

Coughing fits
A tendency to frequent coughing fits when lying down, with a few spells of nightly vomiting, also continues in this age group.

The constipation continues and sometimes even gets worse. How come?

Because children are scared of the painful bowel movements and do everything they can to hold it in. At certain times, when they eventually manage to move their bowels, they cry with pain and sometimes expel a few drops of blood because passing the hard stools opens up a small lesion known as an *anal fissure.*

The child drinks continuously

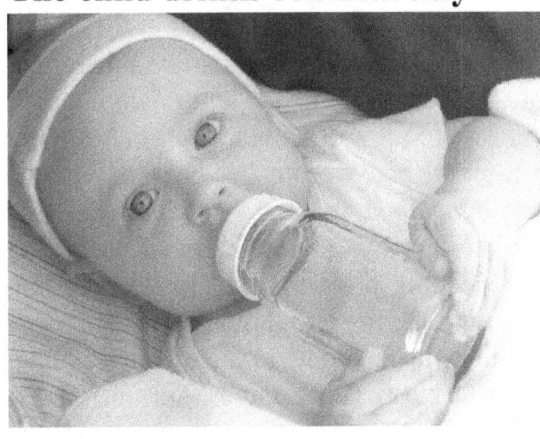

In this second part of their first year, many children with reflux begin to demand a drink continuously.

For example, from when she began to crawl at eight months, my daughter began the habit of always grasping a bottle full of apple juice in her hand. This was the drink of choice to give to babies in the USA at that time. Every now and then she stopped, sat down and drank a little, always producing a very creditable burp immediately afterwards. She demanded a full bottle every evening when she was put down to sleep, so that she could quench her thirst whenever she woke. At that time, we were unaware that *the fact she wanted to drink all the time was a sign that she was tormented by reflux*. It was an instinctive way of giving herself relief, i.e. drinking to force back down the acid she was bringing up. I had not realized that the fluid she was taking was in fact facilitating the reflux, inexorably bringing her gastric contents back up and forcing her to drink again after a short time and perpetuating a vicious cycle.

43

The baby wants to breast feed all the time

When babies are still being breast-fed at this stage, their mothers usually give in and allow them to feed very often, even at night, for the same reason and with the same consequences as the habit of continually drinking a bottle of water.

The baby also regurgitates solid food

It may seem counter-intuitive, but *solid foods* that should by all rights help the baby not to regurgitate *come back up even several hours after a meal. This happens more often with fruit (particularly with blended baby foods) and all other sweet foods,* which accentuate the gastric acid and exacerbate the reflux symptoms.

The baby wakes up all the time

The thing that really worries and exasperates parents most at this stage, however, is *the increasing problem of sleep*. I can illustrate this by describing what happened to Marta. Even though she went down happily, after an hour or two she began to wake up, fidgeting and crying, forcing us to pick her up and comfort her. When we put her back down, she seemed to struggle desperately against a mysterious adversary. She tossed and turned, moaned, lost her dummy, got onto her knees with her bottom in the air (her favourite sleeping position) sat up suddenly and then threw herself down as if she was having a nightmare. Her ceaseless movement almost always meant that she ended up at the other end of her cot, with her head pressed against the bars or cot bumper. This meant that she had no peace, at least until the early hours of the morning. Then she began to sleep more calmly until she eventually woke up to start the day. From time to time, my wife and I were sorely tempted to take her into our bed, and to hell with our good intentions of not spoiling her! I often had to work a night shift at the hospital and the next day was usually real torture. There was no rest.

If the baby gets viral gastroenteritis

In the second six months of life, this possibility is still risky, because when children with reflux contract gastroenteritis, they tend to vomit for longer than other children and their oesophagitis therefore gets much worse. A vicious cycle is therefore set up: the more the baby vomits, the more the tendency to vomit is reinforced.

Sandifer syndrome

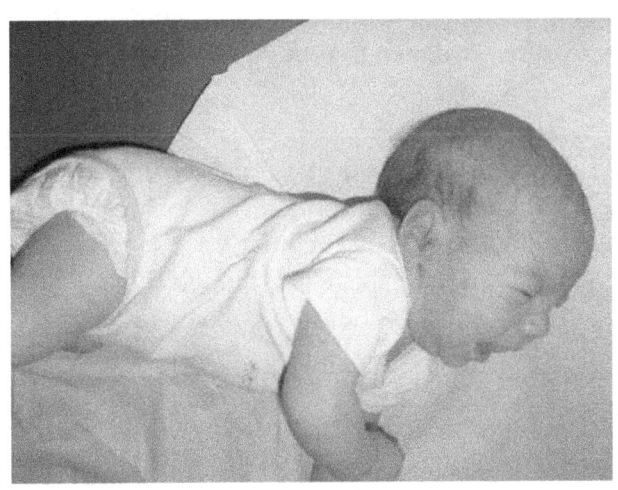

Reflux babies can also be affected by another somewhat unusual condition: *Sandifer syndrome.* The first case I came across, many years ago, was that of baby Sofia, who was brought to see me from Salerno, because her parents were terrified that she had brain damage. She was seven months old and had always suffered from "colic". She constantly regurgitated and woke up screaming 10 times a night, absolutely refusing to lie or even sit down. She seemed a little more settled only if she was picked up constantly and held with her body upright. However, the thing that worried her parents was the fact that for a couple of months *she had been holding her head constantly bent as though she had a stiff neck, and immediately after eating she stiffened all over, throwing her head back*. This prompted her own paediatrician to suggest that she could have a neurological problem. To me it was immediately clear, however, that she was suffering from *Sandifer syndrome* as a consequence of her severe reflux. By instinctively stretching and twisting her neck in that way, she was able to narrow her oesophagus and avoid being affected by acid coming back up from her stomach. Her response to treatment for reflux confirmed that my interpretation was correct. After one week of treatment, Sofia began to hold her head straight. Above all, she stopped being in pain, being unsettled and sleeping badly.

Vagal hyperstimulation with episodes of near-fainting.

The episodes I described under this heading for babies up to six months old can arise at any age, displaying exactly the same development and mechanisms. **Remember that this phenomenon makes the baby *very weak, very pale, as though he or she has fainted. This all happens when the oesophagitis gets worse, often because treatment has been stopped*.**

Episodes of vomiting with blood.

On rare occasions, the oesophagitis is so bad that it causes episodes of vomiting with blood due to *ulceration of the mucosa*. However, even though I have been seeing children with reflux regularly for several decades, I have never come across a case of this kind, though this may be because the children that become my patients are being effectively treated

Can reflux stop children from eating enough?

Among their concerns, parents become anxious that their child is not eating and growing normally because of the reflux. Many end up incorrectly diagnosing reflux in their children because knowledge of its existence is much more widespread nowadays and because some general symptoms can mimic it. For example, I see many mothers blaming this condition for their children's tendency to eat less than expected. However, *it is fairly rare for reflux children not to get enough to eat*. In more than 30 years of experience, I have only come across two or three children who were clearly undernourished due to reflux. And I only ever observed this in children with a malformation known as oesophageal atresia. This happens when part of the oesophagus is missing at birth and the babies have to immediately undergo surgery, which leads to the oesophagus being shortened.

DIAGNOSE REFLUX FROM SIX MONTHS TO ONE YEAR

For this age range too, I base my diagnosis more on the parents' observation of symptoms than on instrumental tests. In other words, I usually do not prescribe an ultrasound or, much less, a pH testing. In any case, babies over six months who come to my attention have usually already had at least one ultrasound scan with results that almost always reflect the same conclusions that can be drawn from the questionnaire. However, there is one difference. *The ultrasound does not measure the intensity of symptoms and the questionnaire is a much better way to determine the entity of the disorder and decide whether and how to treat it.*

WARNING. At this stage, as with the questionnaire designed for babies up to six months of age, in order to confirm reflux, it is essential to detect *the presence of at least one of the symptoms specific to the disorder. These are shown in bold and underlined.*

QUESTIONNAIRE FOR REFLUX FROM SIX MONTHS TO ONE YEAR

1. **When you completed the questionnaire for babies under six months, was the total score 10 with at least one of the highlighted symptoms present?**
   Yes......................3 points
   No..........................0 points

2. **Does your baby still suffer from regurgitation?**
   Rarely....................0 points
   A few times per week... 3 points
   Every day............... 5 points

3. Does your baby experience episodes of projectile vomiting (spontaneous or stimulated by coughing, crying or some other reason)?
Once a week........................2 points
More than once a week...........5 points

4. Does your baby often have hiccups?
Once daily...2 points
Two or more times daily...........................5 points

5. At night does your baby often wake up crying?
at least twice a night...............................2 points
three or more times.........................5 points

6. During the night, does your baby continuously demand water or some other liquid?
once..............................1 point
twice.............................2 points
three or more times.............3 points

7. Does your baby sometimes cry with pain without any reason evident to the paediatrician?
once to twice a week............2 points
three or more times..............3 points

8. Does your baby have spells involving becoming pale and apparently fainting, particularly after regurgitating and vomiting?
Yes...................................5 points
No....................................0 points

9. Does your baby hold his or her neck bent constantly to one side?
Yes...................................3 points
No....................................0 points

10. **<u>Does your baby burp even several hours after a meal?</u>**
every so often...........................0 points
every day.................................3 points

11. **<u>Does your baby find it difficult to swallow small pieces of food that sometimes also trigger bouts of vomiting?</u>**
Every so often....................2 points
Always...............................5 points

12. Does your baby have coughing fits, particularly when lying down, without any symptoms of having a cold?
Every so often..................2 points
Often................................3 points

13. **<u>Does your baby have episodes of vomiting with blood?</u>**
No.....................................0 points
Yes...................................5 points

If your baby **has at least two of the symptoms shown in bold and underlined** and the total score is at least 10 points, it is highly likely that he or she has reflux and you need to see a paediatric gastroen-terologist

TREATING REFLUX FROM SIX MONTHS TO ONE YEAR

What changes after the age of six months to justify changes in the existing treatment?

We have seen that *from 5 to 6 months of age, the reflux becomes less evident because weaning starts with solid foods and the oesophagus lengthens as the child grows*. The amount of acid the baby brings back up remains virtually unchanged, however, and I stress to parents that they must not stop monitoring symptoms and giving treatment despite the apparent "cure". I sympathize with their impatience and desire to stop having to give their child medicines for such long periods. But if they impulsively stop treatment, most of them will soon realize, within about 10 days, that the torment is not over because the symptoms usually return and force them to start treatment again. So, what is the best approach at this stage?

Feeding

After the first six months, it is advisable to continue with breast-feeding, whatever solid foods are gradually introduced. However it might become necessary to stop mother's milk at night, but only if the regurgitation, vomiting and other symptoms get steadily worse despite the drugs. I am well aware that my advice may be at odds with the recommendations of La Leche League experts and lactation consultants, but experience has taught me that it will spare the child (and the mother) a lot of discomfort. *In babies not breast-fed we can give a stage 2 formula* or follow-on formula *thickened exactly as I described for babies up to six months*.

Weaning can continue, though parents should *continue to avoid sweet foods and particularly fruit-based blended baby foods and juices,* for the reasons already explained. However, it is not justified to avoid other foods*, not even tomatoes, which are often advised against without any good reason*.

My remarks about cow's milk-based formula also apply for babies after the age of six months. In particular, if your baby seems to be experiencing more acidity and more discomfort, you can introduce a *soy-based formula. But remember, there is no evidence to support the use of very*

50

expensive hydrolysed formulas, which should be reserved for children with *proven allergies to cow's milk and soy milk.*

Can the child drink when thirsty?

In general, if it is not hot, the water contained in breast milk or thickened milk, combined with the water in food, is enough to satisfy the baby's need for fluids. However, if it is hot or the child still seems thirsty, it is certainly *advisable to offer water, albeit in the form of small and frequent sips. Use a teaspoon, for example or a bottle fitted with a teat with a very small hole.* Children can drink water continuously so that by the end of the day they will have taken enough but without diluting the stomach contents with 30 or more cc all at once, which would promote reflux. On the other hand, *it is not advisable to quench children's thirst with fruit juices or sweetened herbal teas.*

Medicines to be used

The principles I explained for the first six months also apply at this stage. If the child is already being treated with antisecretory agents and antacids, I use the following rule of thumb.

If the symptoms are under control and particularly if the child does not appear to be suffering, *I try to cut out antisecretory agents* (lansoprazole) *by halving the dose. However I continue with antacids*, increasing the dose to 5 ml before each meal and before putting the child down at night. Therefore, if the child is having four or five feeds, I give five or six doses of antacid per day respectively.

If the baby is still showing evident signs of reflux, or if stopping the antisecretory agent worsens the situation, I suggest *continuing or resuming lansoprazole, still giving a 15 mg dose in the morning*, as well as continuing to give antacid at the doses described above for as long as the symptoms require it.

Postural therapy

From the age of six months to one year, many babies with reflux *can benefit from sleeping sitting up*. In this case, however, take great care to ensure that the baby does not slip downward or to the sides as a result of moving while asleep. One of my young patients with severe reflux preferred to sleep *sitting in his stroller* for a couple of years, until his reflux cleared up spontaneously.

Remember that rumours about possible damage to the spine caused by the sitting position are completely unfounded.

In a few months from the release of this edition of the manual, I plan to make available a device which will allow babies up to a year of age to sleep in the position they usually prefer: with their body upright and the head resting on parent's shoulder.

How to manage sleep disorders

This is a crucial subject, because any sleep disorders that may have become established up to this point can cause serious problems for the entire family as well as being a hardship for the baby. *Because of this, I consider the night-time difficulties experienced by reflux babies to represent a true family emergency; a psychosocial problem that needs to be resolved as quickly as possible.*

In my experience, however, an effective and sometimes aggressive treatment can by itself sufficiently limit sleep disorders associated with reflux The main point is to realize that the problem is usually caused by the condition and we have to do everything possible to treat it.

How to treat constipation

If reflux children over six months of age also have *very hard stools that are difficult to expel, the problem can usually be relieved by an aluminium magnesium hydroxide-based antacid (Maalox).* However, if this does not work, *macrogol or lactulose must be used,* following principles similar to those I described with reference to the first few months of age. At this age, the initial dose I recommend is between 10 and 20 ml daily, to be administered in feeds or added to water, yoghurt or other foods, which may be sweetened. Within a few days, the baby should begin to produce softer stools. Now the dose can be increased or decreased according to the results achieved, continuing with the quantity that seems to work best. After a couple of months, these substances can gradually be reduced or discontinued but started again if the constipation comes back, remembering that they are *absolutely harmless and do not cause dependency.*

What should I do if my baby has a cold or cough and the symptoms get worse?
Almost exactly what I described for the first six months of age applies. When the baby has a *cold or cough*, the reflux symptoms tend to get worse even when we are giving treatment that is usually effective. In this situation, I normally advise *topping up treatment with a couple of extra doses of antacid*, to be administered in between meals and at night. I also suggest making more effort with postural therapy, keeping the baby as upright as possible for as long as possible day and night. This approach must be adopted especially for babies attending nurseries, who continually come down with respiratory infections, until they grow out of it.

What should I do if my baby gets gastroenteritis?
Almost exactly what I described for the first six months of age applies in this age group. In this case, there are some essential differences in the measures to implement, because we have usually already started weaning. So, I advise the following:
  a. *Starve the baby completely of solids and liquids* for a few hours, even if he or she seems hungry and thirsty. Do this until the bouts of spontaneous vomiting (vomiting not caused by ingesting anything) come to an end.
  b. Immediately begin to administer *small quantities of antacids* (1 ml every half-hour*)* throughout the first day of the disease (even while the child is still vomiting). During subsequent days, give the antacid more often than usually and use larger amounts than normal.
  c. As soon as the baby stops vomiting, begin to administer teaspoonfuls of *a rehydration salt solution* (various products can be obtained in pharmacies). If the baby finds it distasteful, do not try and force him or her to take it, otherwise the vomiting may get worse. If the baby accepts this solution, carry on for a day or so until the vomiting stops altogether.

d. *If the baby is breast-fed,* breast-feeding can be resumed a couple of hours after the last vomiting episode. *If the baby takes formula milk*, it is better to give only salt solution and not resume feeding until the following day. At this point, it is best to give lactose-free milk, for example a soy-based formula. *If all goes well, on the third day you can go back to the baby's normal milk and normal meals* .

If babies vomit up everything eaten for more than a whole day despite all these measures, particularly if they also have diarrhoea, contact your family paediatrician urgently or go to the emergency room of a paediatric hospital

Diets and medicines for which there is no evidence

On this topic, see my comments for babies under six months of age, which also apply at this stage.

To sum up:

1. *No particular diet,* apart from the precautions regarding sweets and liquids I have already explained
2. *Alginate-based drugs* do not work well in children and it is not worth using them instead of the antacids I've described repeatedly above.

How long will it take for my baby to get better?

When treatment is given, the most evident symptoms usually improve within a few days. A physical improvement does not, however, automatically resolve sleep disorders or the child's habit of wanting to be picked up all the time. Parents need perseverance and courage to overcome these tendencies, with the additional complication that these negative habits are now well-rooted and more difficult to overcome than they were during the first few months.

TREATMENT FAQS

Can antacids cause diarrhoea?

As I said for babies up to 6 months of age, the magnesium hydroxide in antacids can cause some more liquid bowel movements. These may amount to five or six per day. However, this effect is not harmful. Quite the contrary, it helps the baby move its bowels more easily and often helps to resolves the problem of constipation typical of many reflux babies. It also makes it easy to get rid of ingested air, which can be very uncomfortable for reflux babies, as we have seen, and also "colic". So you can ignore this effect altogether unless the baby moves its bowels more than six times per day.

What do I do if my baby gets worse even when being treated?

It is advisable to add one or two doses of antacid per day, between meals if necessary, until your baby is better and then you can go back to the normal regimen.

What happens if my baby doesn't like the taste of the antacid?

Don't get discouraged and give up the treatment if your baby seems not to like the taste of a medicine. It's also not advisable to plough on regardless with the same product, hoping that your baby will accept it eventually, but to try another medicine. For example, if your baby doesn't like Maalox, you could give Riopan or equivalent, whatever available that the baby prefers.

Should I avoid "acid" foods like tomatoes or oranges?

It is not true that slightly more acid foods cause worsening of symptoms. They can therefore be given without any reservations from the first stages of weaning. For obvious reasons, however, it is better not to use the juice of oranges or any other fruit, simply because it is a liquid. This is particularly true if sweetened with any kind of sugar.

My baby is taking much less milk since I began to thicken it. What should I do?

Make sure that the opening in the teat is big enough (star or Y-shaped) to ensure that your baby can suck out the thickened milk without any problems. *Make sure the mixture is not too thick*, it should have a yoghurt -like consistency. *Try with another thickening agent*, for example corn and tapioca flour or carob flour, which can be mixed together. *Don't worry if your baby eats a little less* for a few days. Once he/she gets used to the new flavour, he/she will resume eating and growing as before.

My baby prefers to sleep on its stomach. Should I allow this?

From the age of six months, a baby can usually roll over from lying on its back to lying on its stomach and vice versa. Therefore, b*y the age of six months, the dilemma on how to put your baby down to sleep should no longer be an issue*. In any case, see what I have written on postural therapy for some suggestions on how to put your reflux baby to sleep also at this stage.

How will I know that my child is better?

Sooner or later, nearly all parents of the reflux babies I treat ask me the question: "Will we have to have tests done (ultrasound, pH testing and so on) to see whether we can assume our baby is finally cured?" When the baby seems completely better, many parents decide to stop treatment. They then usually go on to regret this a couple of weeks later when the symptoms come back. I sympathize with their impatience, but unfortunately reflux hardly ever improves permanently before the baby is one year old.

It is better to use a questionnaire for diagnosis under all circumstances. This is even more true when it comes to establishing the severity of the disorder. No instrumental test (from ultrasound to pH testing), however sophisticated, can establish how severe the disorder is at a certain stage more effectively than empirical observation by the parents. *For this purpose, all you have to do is stop treatment for two or three weeks and keep on filling in the relative questionnaire*

CHAPTER IV

REFLUX FROM ONE TO TWO YEARS OF AGE

By the time children have reached the age of one, very few of them can truly be considered "cured" of reflux

This small proportion will be made up of children with a particularly mild form of the condition. In this case, all treatment can be stopped, including precautions over sweet foods and liquids. *Most of the other reflux children will continue to experience the disorder, albeit usually to a lesser extent*.

The first thing that happens, as the months go by, is that the *reflux becomes less constant than before*. In other words, it sometimes disappears altogether for a while, then all the symptoms suddenly recur, to confound the parents and even the paediatrician. *In particular, if we stop treatment, some of the symptoms remain unchaged, and are joined by some new symptoms more characteristic of this stage*.

The following symptoms usually remain:

Hiccupping

Hiccups *reappear more sporadically*, but sometimes last all day.

Tendency to drink continually.

Some reflux children, however, show an opposite trend. They drink very little, as though they realize that fluids make them more uncomfortable.

Waking up continuously.

This symptom is almost always present and is the one that causes most discomfort and suffering to the child and the family. The waking is caused by a burning feeling due to the oesophagitis and the sensation of choking, sometimes caused by acid coming back up towards the mouth. *Unsettled sleep, continuous movement from one side of the cot to the other, babies sleeping on their knees with their heads resting on the bed and their bottoms in the air.* I remember watching my daughter rolling from one side of the bed to other as though possessed. I thought at the time that she behaved like this due to her temperament (very lively!). Only much later, after talking to the parents of many children with reflux, did I realize that those sudden jerking movements helped protect against the threat of acid reflux.

Because the sleep of reflux babies is so disturbed, in daytime they often *appear tired and tense.*

Retching and vomiting when eating food in pieces. Dysphagia of reflux.

Many children with reflux, up to the age of two or more, refuse to eat solid food cut up (even if it is in very small bits). When they try to swallow this sort of food they react retching or even vomiting. It is pointless trying to persuade or force them to swallow food that is not blended or sieved, concerned that they will "never learn to eat properly". Their refusal is no mere whim but a sign of oesophagitis. It will only go away when they are two years old or more and the inflammation improves spontaneously. However, as we will see, this "dysphagia", a further very common symptom of reflux, may reappear also much later, even in adolescence, whenever the reflux flares up strongly for some reason.

Coughing at night
This symptom reappears periodically in children with reflux, particularly when the condition gets out of control. If the child has already started to attend nursery, it will be difficult to establish whether the cough is due to reflux or to the recurrent viral respiratory infections that the child contracts coming in contact with other children. *In any case, whatever its cause, a cough facilitates reflux and reflux facilitates coughing.* This may set up a vicious cycle that could last for months.

Vagal hyperstimulation with near-fainting spells..
The spells I described for younger children under this heading can recur at any age. Whenever the child's reflux-induced oesophagitis is very intense (even if this is not immediately evident), he or she may suddenly go pale, break out in a cold sweat and go floppy with a pained expression, seeming almost to faint.

Constipation

Constipation continues, albeit sporadically. Towards two years of age, this symptom can actually get more pronounced, presenting itself with *"stool holding spells"*. I.e. the child starts suddenly screaming with pain feeling at the same time the very strong urge to go and the impulse of doing everything to avoid passing the stools. To give you an idea of what these children go through in these instances, here what one of them said to me: "Doctor Albani, my "cacca" has thorns…"

Episodes of vomiting with blood.

Very rarely, when a child with reflux remains untreated for a long time, the oesophageal mucosa becomes ulcerated and the child may vomit blood.

The following symptoms, that could also be from other conditions, appear or get worse as the child approaches two years of age .

Bad breath

One of my daughter's symptoms that I could never explain at the time was bad breath. I thought it was due to a gum infection or sinusitis. Later on, as I saw more and more children with reflux, it became evident that in these children the halitosis is caused by acidified food going back up into the oesophagus, particularly at night when the child lies horizontal. This symptom is so much more common in reflux children that it can be considered a classic sign of it, usually persisting into adulthood.

Recurrent vomiting.

Regurgitation is unlikely to still be present in children who have passed their first birthday. However, whenever the reflux flares up, *vomiting* becomes more frequent, particularly at night when the reflux is more intense. These relapses are usually triggered by other problems, such as a respiratory tract infection with cough, viral gastroenteritis or the imminent eruption of a tooth.

Intractable vomiting episodes

During these episodes, children may continue vomiting for several days at a time, often immediately after going down with viral gastroenteritis. If they are not treated quickly and effectively, *they can end up in hospital, dehydrated and malnourished*, having not been unable to take any foods and liquids for days on end.

"Tummy ache"

When reflux children are nearly two years old and able to put things more effectively in words, they often complain of a *"tummy ache*, pointing to the *middle of their abdomen near their belly button, or above it right at their stomach level*. This is usually a sign that the oesophagitis has gotten worse, even when the child indicates a point of his tummy that seems to suggest a bowel problem.

Refusal to eat breakfast.

These children often go through phases when *they eat less than usual*, *refusing* in particular *to eat breakfast*, because they wake up with an upset stomach due to the worsening of reflux in the lying position.

Can reflux stop children from eating enough and growing?

Since I get a continuous stream of questions about this, I believe it is essential to repeat the unequivocal answer I gave with regard to younger children. Instead of concentrating on treating the discomfort that the reflux causes to their children, many parents are terrified by the possibility that they will not grow properly or that they will develop severe dietary deficiencies.

I never tire of saying that it is very rare for reflux children not to eat enough because of their disorder. For the umpteenth time, I have only seen two or three cases of malnutrition in children with reflux in all my decades of experience. However, these cases were always young children who underwent surgery at birth due to a malformation known as oesophageal atresia i.e. a congenital abnormality in which part of the oesophagus is missing.

DIAGNOSIS OF REFLUX FROM ONE TO TWO YEARS OF AGE

At this stage too, the best way to diagnose reflux is *observing the symptoms and fill in the relevant questionnaire* for this age. As usual, for reflux to be suspected in a child, *the symptoms must include at least one of those shown underlined and in bold*. To be more certain, it is always advisable to fill in also the questionnaires for previous stages. *If the scores (the score relevant to the age and the previous scores) exceed 10, the child is almost certainly suffering from reflux* and in this case it is advisable to consult a gastroenterologist for a definitive diagnosis and treatment.

QUESTIONNAIRE FOR REFLUX FROM ONE TO TWO YEARS OF AGE

1. **Did your child suffer from reflux symptoms before his or her first birthday?**
   (For this purpose, fill in the previous questionnaires)
   Yes = 5 points
   No = 0 points
2. As your child approached the age of two and became old enough to explain, did he or she complain of stomach-ache (pointing to the stomach area)?
   Once weekly........................2 points
   Twice or more ....3 points

3. **Does your child have bad breath in the morning?**
   Sporadically.....................2 points
   Often...........................5 points

4. **Does your child often have hiccups?**
   Once weekly.................0 points
   Three times weekly............2 points
   Many times a week.............3 points

5. Does your child refuse to eat breakfast?
   Sporadically................0 points
   Twice weekly...................2 points
   Three or more times........3 points

6. **Does your child vomit periodically for no identifiable reason?**
   Once weekly.............................2 points
   More than once weekly...........5 points

7. **Does your child vomit if he or she has a cough, cries a lot, goes on a car trip etc.?**
   Sporadically................2 points
   Often............................5 points

8. **Does your child have intractable vomiting attacks that last for several days?**
   No................................0 points
   Yes................................5 points

9. Does your child still refuse food cut up small and prefer pureed food?
   No................................0 points
   Yes................................2 points

10. Does your child carry around a bottle containing water or other fluid
    and continuously drink from it?
    No............................. .....0 points
    Yes................................2 points

11. Does your child wake up frequently with night fears?
    Wakes up twice..............................3 points
    Wakes up twice or more...................5 points

12. Does your child drink at night when he or she wakes up?
Once.................................1 point
twice...............................2 points
Three or more times...........................3 points

13. **Does your child suffer from spells when he/she becomes pale and seems to faint, particularly after regurgitating or vomiting?**
Yes..................................5 points
No...................................0 points

14. Does your child often refuse to eat breakfast?
Yes..................................2 points
No...................................0 points

TREATING REFLUX FROM ONE TO TWO YEARS OF AGE

If the reflux is mild

Because mild forms of the condition can disappear altogether after one year of age, *treatment can be stopped for good in some children*. However, you have to be prepared to start again after a few weeks' break, if your child begins to vomit frequently, sleep very badly and hiccup after many feedings. *The most reasonable strategy for these children is to alternate periods when you do not take any precautions with periods when you return to the treatment described above.*

In more serious forms of reflux, when the relative questionnaire score is well over 10, *it is often necessary to give antisecretory agents periodically.* For example, during flare-ups, I personally prescribe lansoprazole for two or three weeks at a time if intense symptoms come back.

And in such cases *antacids (Maalox, Riopan or Gadral) must be administered regularly in five 5 ml doses daily*, prior to meals and before going to sleep at night, *or in three 10 ml doses, one in the morning, one in the afternoon and one before going to sleep.*

If the reflux continues at significant levels

Stopping treatment brings about a rapid deterioration of conditions for the great majority of children who have experienced reflux during their first year of life. So *they usually have to resume treatment and continue with few breaks until they are at least two years old.*

Many parents can't wait to stop all the drugs and forget about reflux forever, but many others are reluctant to stop treatment for even one day, in fear of doing unknown damage. No worry, the only consequence of making a mistake fuelled by over-optimism is that the child will suffer a little for a few days and this can be easily remedied by re-introducing treatment. Let's take a look at what treatment changes are required compared to the previous stage.

Diet

In my opinion, *whether they are reflux sufferers or not, by the time they are one, children should have tried every food the parents eat, including seafood, shellfish, hot peppers, pasta sauce and so on*. If they like it and are able to swallow small pieces of food, they can eat these foods regularly instead of the blended baby foods they ate during previous months or, if they prefer, they can alternate the two.

The things that continue to pose a few problems to reflux children are *liquid foods (such as unthickened milk, clear soup etc.) and sweet foods, which should be avoided as far as possible*. At breakfast time, they can dunk a couple of rusks in their milk, which is better thickened with one of the flour agents used during the first year of life.

Water can be offered freely, provided you usually follow the principle of making them take small sips.

Postural therapy

Children aged between one and two years of age should also *use any method that allows them to sleep with their bodies as upright as possible*. Children can use reclining seats, wedge cushions or even baby buggies if they show clearly that they prefer to sleep in this position and manage to rest better, without any interruptions. However, *if children prefer to lie down, even on their stomachs, there is no reason to force them to do otherwise.*

How to manage sleep disorders

Usually, if the reflux is properly treated, waking up and unsettled sleep are less of a problem at this age. However, many children have become so used to getting attention during the night because of the reflux they suffered during their first year of life that they still wake up all the time even though the treatment is effective. Effective treatment means all the dietary measures I have described so far, the administration of antacids and antisecretory agents and postural therapy. In this case, I explain to parents that the waking up at night is no longer linked to the discomfort caused by reflux and they can take a firmer approach without having to feel too guilty.

How long will it take for my child to get better?

If children with reflux have never been treated before their first birthday, effective treatment usually improves symptoms within a few days or one week at most. Children are able to rest more effectively and show no more signs of pain or discomfort. They no longer vomit and generally appear more content. Among other things, this clear improvement confirms that the diagnosis was correct. Conversely, if the reported symptoms do not clear up at all following treatment, the diagnosis is very likely to have been incorrect and the child has simply developed some unfortunate habits due to the conditioning received in previous months.

How to treat constipation

Constipation usually reflects the progress of the reflux and will improve without further measures if the reflux is properly treated. However, if children continue to have very hard stools and withhold them for a long time despite taking antacids, it is best to give something to soften the stools. As with younger children, I use lactulose or macrogol for this purpose. For this age group, I prescribe two or three dessert spoonful's per day, to be added to milk, yoghurt or water etc. In this case too, I advise continuing this regimen for a few months to help the child forget their experience of painful bowel movements and break their habit of avoiding going to the toilet.

What happens if the child has a cough and cold

As previously stated, *the arrival of a cold, particularly if accompanied by a cough, can cause an exacerbation or return of the reflux.* So, it is best to be prepared to step up treatments, increasing the number of antacid doses and always administering antacid after specific vomiting episodes.

If the child has gastroenteritis

In the case of children with a more severe form of reflux, the tendency to vomit indefinitely after a gastroenteritis persists into their second year and beyond. The measures I advise to prevent or treat this intractable vomiting are the same described for the previous age group.

Firstly, *complete fasting*, without even taking fluids, for some hours following the onset of the repeated vomiting episodes. Then, *very frequent administration of small doses of antacid* (for example, 2 ml of Maalox, Riopan or Gadral every half-hour) for at least one whole day. When the child has stopped being sick for two or three hours, start giving *a salt solution for rehydration*, or frequent sips of water if the child refuses the rehydration solution. It is best to give these fluids cold from the refrigerator, because this has a slight anti-nausea effect. Lastly, once vomiting has subsided for at least a whole day, re-introduce the usual diet, in small frequent meals, avoiding cow's milk and dairy products for one more day.

Diets and medicines for which there is no evidence

Some of my colleagues insistently claim that reflux can be due to *a dietary allergy or intolerance* and often put reflux babies on a diet, but I stress with equal insistence that *there is no evidence to support this practice*. If I happen to see a child who has been treated in this way, I always advise the parents to stop any diet and start the treatment I have described. The inevitable outcome is that the child immediately improves and is delighted to go back to eating banned foods, as are the parents.

REFLUX TREATMENT FAQs

What happens if children refuse solid food until they are two?
I repeat what I have already said for younger children: *reflux children refuse to eat solid food because their oesophagitis makes swallowing more difficult*. They are not being fussy, even though this might seem the case. This problem may crop up now and then in subsequent years, depending on the intensity of the oesophagitis. Appropriate treatment of the reflux greatly reduces or eliminates this kind of dysphagia.

My child has been better since she started taking antacid, but now she has diarrhoea...
Remember: magnesium hydroxide in the antacids can cause up to five or six liquid stools a day. However, this effect is not associated with any risk of damage. Quite the contrary, it helps children to resolve the

constipation problem typical of many reflux babies. It also makes it easy to get rid of ingested air, which is very uncomfortable for reflux children, as we have seen.

It's best to add one or two doses of antacid between meals for a few days until your child is better and then you can go back to the normal doses.

My child doesn't like the taste of the antacid and spits it all out
If the child shows distaste for or is fed up of taking one of the medicines, try not to get discouraged to the point of giving up treatment, or the symptoms might return. It's also pointless to carry on with the same product, because you may end up making your child even more reluctant to accept any medication. Instead, if your child doesn't like Maalox, try with Riopan, or Gadral, which may be more palatable to her/him. In the end you'll always be able to find a product that your child will take without too much fuss.

Should I avoid "acid" foods like tomatoes or oranges?
Remember that slightly more acid fruit doesn't cause more acidity. For obvious reasons, however, it is better not to use large glasses of juice of oranges or any other fruit, simply because they are liquids. This is particularly true if sweetened with any kind of sugar.

CHAPTER V

REFLUX FROM TWO YEARS OF AGE TO ADOLESCENCE

Early in my career as a medical writer, a few years after I returned from the united States, I began to answer letters sent to the magazine *Io e il mio Bambino* [My baby and me]. These letters were often written by despairing mothers asking for advice. After a couple of years doing this job, I analysed the hundreds of requests I had received by that time and realized that the great majority concerned one specific problem:
"My child won't sleep".

My second finding was that the period when all these children were unable to sleep was usually limited to the first two and a half years of life. I rarely received letters from the parents of older children with the same problem. My subsequent experience allowed me to get to the bottom of the statistics. I realized that ***90 per cent of sleep disorders in younger children are linked to gastroesophageal reflux and the problem tails off after two years of age because the reflux also diminishes significantly at this age***. However, a good proportion of children continue to exhibit reflux symptoms well beyond this limit and some are even destined to have the problem into adulthood. After the age of two, the situation nevertheless changes in such a way that the problem risks going undetected and untreated even though various signals show that it continues causing a good deal of discomfort. Let's look at what actually happens.

Halitosis

Because reflux was little-known at the beginning of my career, I didn't realize that my daughter's **bad breath** was **one of its most telling signs**. So, in her case I forced her to clean her teeth three times a day, but to little avail.

Recurrent stomach-ache

After two years of age, children begin to be able to describe the pain they experience from time to time as "stomach-ache". They touch themselves in the epigastric area, immediately below the ribs. The pain mainly makes itself felt early in the morning or a couple of hours after breakfast and then comes and goes without following any particular pattern.

Refusal to eat breakfast
This habit is due to nausea and a sensation that the stomach is "closed" at awakening, linked to the fact that reflux gets worse at night, when gastric acid can come back up more easily due to lying horizontally.

Poor appetite
I have found that poor appetite coincides with periods when the condition is more active. A word of caution: this will not cause malnutrition or stunted growth because children always make up for it on days (or at the times of day) when they feel better.

Vagal hyperstimulation episodes
These are spells when the child almost seems to faint. They occur in direct proportion to the number of episodes experienced previously. One day, a five-year old patient of mine named Pietro scared his parents so much with one of these near-fainting episodes that he ended up in hospital and underwent a round of testing by cardiologists and neurologists, who found nothing abnormal. In this case too, as I regularly see happen, his parents had underestimated his reflux and stopped treating him for a few months, thinking (or hoping) that the condition had permanently cleared up.

Cough and laryngospasm and/or bronchial spasm
Remember that, as with younger children, once children have passed their second birthday, there is a *close relationship between coughing caused by respiratory infections and exacerbation of the reflux.* Many children with reflux may experience episodes of *bronchial spasm*, when they struggle to breathe and make a wheezy sound as though they were having an asthma attack, or *laryngospasm,* when their cough sounds like a seal bark and their breathing is very raucous.

Vomiting with blood.

If the esophagitis has been neglected for a long time, ulceration of the mucosa may develop. This may bleed and cause vomiting with blood. Fortunately, the symptom is so rare in children that I've never even seen one case.

Constipation

The problem of constipation *culminates at around the age of two* and often leads children to withhold their stools to avoid the pain of passing very hard faeces (stool with thorns!). For this fear, some children can go several days without having a bowel movement and frequently twist around and squeeze their buttocks trying as best they can to resist the urge. The resulting vicious cycle risks going on indefinitely. As I already explained in the case of younger children, effective treatment of reflux usually puts paid to this problem as well. Otherwise, I advise administering *lactulose or macrogol* (two or three desertspoonfuls daily) for a few months. These substances soften the stools and make them much easier to pass. As time goes on, the vicious cycle described is permanently broken, without side effects or the risk of forming a habit.

Quality of sleep and dreams

The most evident sleep disturbances, when children wake up crying and calling for their parents to pick them up and comfort them, tend to wane at this stage. However, if the child still has significant reflux after this age, *bedtime may be somewhat disturbed by acid coming up* and *interrupting sleep patterns*.

Example: at about three years of age, my daughter began to experience episodes when she sat up in bed, often with her eyes open, but in a state of sleeping wakefulness during which it was clear that she was in the grip of a *nightmare*. She sometimes even sleepwalked. All these effects are referred to as parasomnias and often attributed to psychological disorders that are not properly identified. In my experience, these very distressing experiences are usually linked with the sensation of choking caused by acid reflux. Children who experience such nightmares frequently are often scared of going to bed in the evening and suffer from **anxiety and melancholia**.

Some case histories are given below.

Examples of children with sleep disorders
Hans, Angela, Simone and Matteo

I have a very vivid memory of a six-year-old boy named **Hans,** who was brought to me because he was suffering from **intractable vomiting**. The problem had been going on for weeks. The poor child was unable to eat normally and had ben vomiting at least a couple of times a day, to the point of having lost 5 kg in the past three weeks. *Hans immediately struck me as very scared and depressed, as if he had lost hope*. He told me that *he couldn't sleep properly any more and that he had horrible dreams and was scared of dying.*

Proper anti-reflux treatment was all it took to help him put the weight back on in a couple of weeks. Above all, he went back to being a happy child with undisturbed dreams.

Another young nine-year-old patient of mine named *Angela* was bought to see me because she had been unable to sleep for months. *She was scared of going to bed because she feared being suffocated in her sleep "by thieves or murderers"*. Her parents had taken her to a psychologist, but to no avail. As soon as I saw her, I remembered that she had suffered from gastroesophageal reflux until she was two and this had then apparently cleared up. I immediately realized that she still had very revealing symptoms of the condition: she often had bad breath, hiccups, some difficulty in swallowing food and sporadic episodes of vomiting that could not otherwise be explained. In Angela's case too, good anti-reflux therapy worked much better and faster than the psychotherapy she had undergone.

Eight-year old *Simone* was brought to see me after much shunting to and fro between specialists because he had bad headache as well as frequent morning vomiting. He had even undergone tests to rule out a brain tumour. He hadn't been able to sleep properly for months. Nightmares woke him and he kept ending up in his parents' bed. They allowed him to do this even though they were as tired out as him by the broken nights. His mother often had to pick him up from school because he would get sudden stomach-aches. The bad breath that everyone had written off as a simple problem of oral hygiene was his other prevailing symptom. It goes without saying that the child had been put by other doctors on a special diet for months due to supposed "food intolerances", without any result. A few days after starting my anti-reflux treatment, Simone began to rest properly and stopped vomiting. His mother commented, "we've got our lives back"…

A lean and athletic 14-year-old boy named *Matteo* came to see me because *he could no longer eat pieces of meat, as he was terrified of choking when he swallowed them.* He showed great promise at football and was attending a football academy, but lately he had lost a lot of weight and did not have any energy for the training sessions. He also *hardly slept and had "terrible" dreams*. Recently, he had also been having full-blown *panic attacks*. He had been receiving treatment from a neuropsychiatrist for this reason but without great success. He spoke monosyllabically in a tired, worried tone. He seemed demoralized and sceptical of finding a solution to his problem, which had affected him for months and been described by other doctors as psychosomatic. He had begun to believe he was really going mad and was a hopeless case. However, his history immediately made me suspect his was a case of gastroesophageal reflux that had always been overlooked and never treated. In this case too, treatment for the physical condition helped to quickly restore his taste for food, his energies and his mental balance.

DIAGNOSING REFLUX FROM TWO YEARS OLD TO ADOLESCENCE

QUESTIONNAIRE FROM TWO YEARS OLD TO ADOLESCENCE

1. **<u>Did your child experience reflux symptoms when younger? (complete the relevant questionnaires).</u>**
   Yes = 5 points
   No = 0 points

2. **<u>Does your child have pains, burning or spasms at the stomach entrance?</u>**
   Sporadically.....................0 points
   Often............................3 points
   Usually...........................5 points

3. **<u>Does your child vomit from time to time without being apparently ill</u>**
   Once a month.....................2 points
   More than once a month.........3 points

4. **<u>Does your child have bad breath, especially in the morning?</u>**
   Sporadically.....................0 points
   Often............................5 points
   Usually..........................7 points

5. **<u>Does your child have the sensation of a bitter fluid coming back up into the mouth?</u>**
   Sporadically...............0 points
   Usually......................5 points

6. **<u>Does your child often have considerable difficulty in swallowing solid foods?</u>**
   No..............................0 points
   Yes.............................5 points

7. Does your child prefer not to eat breakfast because of an upset stomach?
   No...............................0 points
   Usually.....................3 points

8. Does your child suffer from abdominal pains that cannot be other-wise explained?
   a few times a month.....2 points
   many times a month.....3 points

9. Is he or she constipated?
   Sporadically................0 points
   Usually..........................3 points

10. Does your child refuse to eat breakfast due to "stomach-ache"?
    Sporadically.....................0 points
    Often..............................2 points
    Usually..........................3 points

11. **Does your child experience spells when he or she becomes very pale and sick and collapses as though about to faint**?
    No................................0 points
    Yes...............................5 points

12. Does your child get carsick or seasick?
    Once a year....................0 points
    2-3 times a year..........2 points
    Every time...............3 points

13. Does your child have a cough only at night, without symptoms of respiratory disorders?
    Sporadically................0 points
    Usually..........................3 points

14. Does your child have attacks of bronchospasm that cannot be explained by allergic asthma? Sporadically....................0 points Often...........................3 points
15. Does your child wake up feeling anxious at night? Sporadically...............0 points Usually........................5 points
16. Does he or she drink at night when awake? Rarely..........................0 points Often............................2 points Usually........................3 points As usual, when interpreting the questionnaire results, beware of jumping to hasty conclusions. ***Unless you have recorded at least two of the symptoms show underlined and in bold, there is no reason to suspect reflux***. If you have entered two or more of the highlighted symptoms and scored more than 10 on the questionnaire, your child probably, still has significant reflux and should therefore be treated by a specialist.

What if the problem is caused by Helicobacter?

An infection caused *by Helicobacter pylori*, bacteria can become estab-

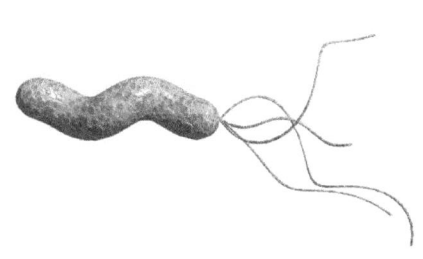

lished in the stomach mucosa and cause chronic inflammation. This phenomenon may even lead to a gastric or duodenal ulcer over time. It has nothing to do with reflux but may be mistaken for the condition because it often causes epigastric pain and can be accompanied by excessive vomiting, sometimes with blood.

However, it must be remembered that *whereas reflux is a very common problem, Helicobacter infection is very unusual in children.*

Helicobacter can also usually be distinguished from reflux by certain characteristics.

1. *It never starts as early in life as reflux*, but only once the early years have passed

2. *It does not occur with regurgitation and signs of oesophagitis: hiccupping, swallowing difficulty, vagal hyperstimulation spells and so on.* If you have lingering doubts, *stool and blood tests give an initial provisional confirmation of the disease, while endoscopy of the oesophagus, stomach and duodenum allow a firm diagnosis*. Endoscopy shows inflammation *in the stomach* (which is never present with reflux) and the specialist can take small *biopsies* that reveal the presence of the bacterium directly when examined under the microscope.

TREATING REFLUX FROM TWO YEARS OF AGE TO ADOLESCENCE

Stop the treatments if symptoms disappear

Because reflux disappears or becomes inconstant and intermittent in a good proportion of child sufferers from two years of age onwards, it is reasonable to try and discontinue all treatments and monitor the situation, maintaining a certain level of vigilance.

Resume the treatments if symptoms reappear

In approximately 50 per cent of cases, the disorder will reappear sooner or later often a couple of weeks after stopping the drugs but often months later when the problem has apparently gone away for good. In this case, *if the symptoms (repeated vomiting, bad breath, hiccupping and sleep disorders) persist, it is best to resume treatment.*

The fundamental principles of treatment remain the same:

1. *drink water in small, frequent sips and cut out or at least limit sweet things. Apart from this, children/adolescents should be able to eat everything they want, including hot peppers.*
2. *take an antisecretory agent like lansoprazole,* 15 -30 mg according to body weight, in the morning.
3. *take an aluminium and magnesium hydroxide or magaldrate-based antacid,* one tablespoonful (approximately 15 ml) three or four times daily with the last dose taken just before going to bed in the evening.

Treatment duration

When treatment is resumed, it should not take the form of a few doses here and there when symptoms occur, but last for at least three or four weeks, because the symptoms reveal the presence of *oesophagitis* and an appropriate period of acidity control is needed to treat it.

If children/adolescents experience frequent symptom recurrences, in addition to giving full courses of treatment as described, it is a good idea *to give a regular antacid, at least in the evening before going to bed.*

If the child has gastroenteritis

The tendency to vomit endlessly after gastroenteritis may also continue after the age of two. The measures I advise to prevent or treat this intractable vomiting are as described for the previous age group.

1. Firstly, *complete fasting, without even taking fluids, for some hours* after the onset of the repeated vomiting episodes.

2. At the same time, start *very frequent administration of small doses (2 ml) of an antacid (Maalox plus, Mylanta, Riopan), which should be continued* for at least one full day.

3. *In the meantime*, when the child/adolescent *has not been sick for at least two or three hours, he or she can sip cold water or Coca-Cola or even suck ice cubes.*

4. *When you are sure that the vomiting has stopped for several hours (6-7 hours)*, the child of adolescent can start to eat small meals, if hungry, avoiding cow's milk and dairy products for at least one day.

5. *After each of these episodes, treatment must be continued as described for children/adolescents who start to vomit again months/years after ending treatment.*

Can reflux be cured permanently by surgery?

It could be advisable for adolescents who often present with severe painful symptoms, blood in the vomit, severe swallowing difficulties and so on to undergo more invasive investigations (such as esophagoscopy) to discover any oesophageal erosions and ulcers) and consider surgery to correct the defect. Several decades ago, Nissen invented a surgical technique known as *"fundoplication"* and this usually resolves the problem. The reasons why this operation is only carried out rarely are:

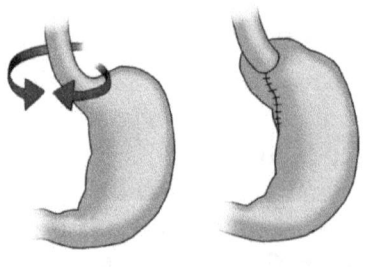

1. It is an invasive operation requiring a general anaesthetic.

2. The operation might not achieve the intended purpose (this happens in approximately 10 per cent of cases).

3. It might have side effects, such as not being able to burp or vomit even in situations where vomiting is a necessary defence mechanism.
For this reason, the operation is only indicated in very severe situations that do not respond satisfactorily to medical treatment.

How is constipation treated?

The problem of constipation is at its worse from the age of two to three, when children tend to avoid going to the toilet for several days at a time. It should be treated with determination to prevent it from becoming a vicious cycle: *if the stools are hard, the child becomes terrified of feeling pain and tends to avoid going to the toilet at all costs, so stools get even harder.* In children under six, treatment should be given without the child being aware of it to avoid rebellion and resistance. It involves administering two or three desertspoonfuls (15 ml) of lactulose or macrogol (no side effects and no habit forming) daily for five to six months. This long-term treatment makes the child forget the experience of painful bowel movements. Remember that the vicious cycle may begin again if treatment is stopped too soon.

Managing sleep disorders

In my experience, sleep disorders experienced from the age of two, "parasomnias" during which children have waking nightmares and often sleepwalk, are strongly linked to the recurrence of reflux. *So, I consider the appearance or exacerbation of these symptoms to be a good reason for resuming treatment for reflux as described in previous sections.*

Pointless diets and medicines

As before, there is no evidence that diets prescribed for alleged "intolerances" do reflux any good, even throughout this long age range. Avoiding cow's milk and dairy products at least temporarily may be useful during symptom flare-ups, because milk is a liquid and needs a lot of acid to digest it, as I have repeatedly said.

CHAPTER VI

REFLUX IN ADULTS

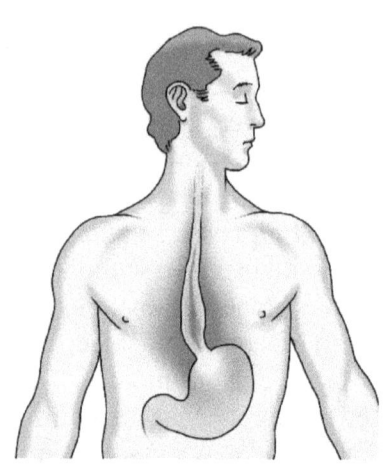

In the USA, it is calculated that 20 per cent of the adult population regularly suffers from *heartburn, which is a burning sensation at the stomach level.* In the past, those who experienced it usually interpreted it as a sign of "gastritis" or "poor digestion". In recent decades, it has become clear that in most cases heartburn is a sign of reflux oesophagitis and this condition is much more common than other similar disorders such as gastritis and ulcer. *Often the burning sensation is not restricted to the stomach entrance but extends upward into the thorax towards the throat.*

Acid regurgitation

The other symptom that is always present is acid regurgitation, which does not usually reach the mouth. This acid reflux is always clearly discernible as a bitter fluid coming up into the throat and immediately being swallowed back down, with a sense of distaste.

Food intolerances?

During this regurgitation, reflux sufferers can recognize the taste of food ingested during the previous meal. If one of the ingredients has a particularly strong flavour (such as peppers or garlic) sufferers often *blame that food for their "poor digestion". So they* start avoiding it mistakenly *believing that they have developed an intolerance to that particular food,* even though in the past they have not noticed any problem with it.

Build-up of wind and burping
The stomachs and abdomens of sufferers are often full of air. This gives them a sensation that they are not digesting properly and that their food "is lying on their stomach".

Hiccupping
Sufferers hiccup much more often than others. The hiccups can last all day and sometimes none of the usual tricks works (such as holding your breath, pushing your stomach out and holding your nose, swallowing a few drops of lemon, etc.).

Difficulty getting off to sleep and frequent awakenings at night
In the evening, after dinner, reflux sufferers find it very difficult to go to sleep in a horizontal position and often drop off more easily sitting up in an armchair than lying down, waiting until very late to go to bed.

Tendency to drink at night
Once in bed, acidity will wake reflux sufferers frequently and cause a burning sensation that triggers a desire to drink. They inevitably take a bottle of water to bed and keep it within easy reach on their bedside table and *drink a lot several times a night*. The more they drink, however, the more the stomach contents come back up and make them want to drink more. So this habit often ends up being counterproductive.

Coughing at night
At night, reflux sufferers often have a cough and sometimes wake up with a feeling of suffocation. These symptoms are caused by acid coming back up into contact with the larynx with the risk of going down into the trachea.

Bad breath
In the morning, they usually wake with a furred tongue and bad breath, no matter how diligently they cleaned their teeth and tongue the previous evening. The same effect occurs in the daytime, after taking a nap, when

they often wake up with a furred tongue, a bad breath and a feeling of indigestion.

Swallowing difficulties

At certain times, swallowing suddenly becomes difficult. Mouthfuls of food get stuck halfway down the oesophagus and cause a painful spasms that forces sufferers to stop eating and wait for the sensation to pass. These spasms can sometimes culminate in a *feeling that the throat is very tight or closing*. When combined with the swallowing difficulty, this causes sufferers to avoid food, particularly solid food, for fear of choking.

Oesophageal colic

Violent oesophageal colic causes such acute pain in the centre of the chest that sometimes it mimics a heart attack.

Vagal hyperstimulation

Vagal hyperstimulation attacks can occur independently of or, more frequently, at the same time as oesophageal colic. This means that from time to time the pain is accompanied or followed by a near-fainting episode. This naturally makes the sufferer even more worried and may cause a full-blown panic attack.

Vomiting with blood

The possibility of this symptom occurring is much greater in adults than in children, because the damaging action of acid in the oesophagus has sometimes gone on for years without proper treatment. The onset of this sign is usually accompanied by oesophageal colic and vagal hyperstimulation attacks. As the patient gets older, in such cases it is more likely he/she will develop Barrett's oesophagus.

Constipation

Constipation may continue, although in adults it does not cause the discomfort and fear typical of the early years.

Pregnancy, obesity and reflux:

Very many women *suffer severe reflux throughout most of their pregnancies, particularly during the second part*. The uterus presses against the abdominal organs to push the stomach upward, promoting the onset of hiatus hernia and therefore reflux.

For similar reasons, *the same thing happens to people who are overweight and, worse still, obese.*

The stories of Mara and Giulia

The story of a young patient of mine named *Mara* is a good illustration of just how much gastroesophageal reflux can affect a person's physical and mental health. Mara came to see me because she was at her wit's end and could not stand her situation any longer.

While convalescing from open-heart surgery, some very disturbing symptoms had suddenly appeared a few months previously. She experienced *a constant burning sensation in her chest*, behind her sternum, that got worse an hour or two after eating and that she initially thought was due to the surgery wound. *She also vomited from time to time. In addition, she could not swallow properly*, so that *food would get blocked halfway down her chest*. This made her feel increasingly scared and she eventually started eating much less than usual. This made her lose a lot of weight and she seemed to be embarking on a very dangerous downward spiral. *She experienced painful spasms* in the centre of her chest, accompanied by *bradycardia* (very slow heart rate). The heart surgeon was unable to explain this phenomenon; the surgery had gone extremely well and there was no theoretical reason for this to happen. She was already under a lot of strain, having to undergo open-heart surgery, so her new symptoms made her become deeply depressed. As it often happens in similar situations, her condition triggered panic attacks that stopped her going out and doing things. She was in a real mess.

It seemed obvious to me that Mara had begun to suffer from severe oesophagitis from gastroesophageal reflux, perhaps as a complication of the surgery she had undergone. This was the obvious (to me) cause of the burning sensation, vomiting, swallowing difficulties and painful spasms. Also the bradycardia, in my view, could be explained as one of the effects of the oesophagitis, as a sign of the vagal hyperstimulation I have repeatedly mentioned.

Mara's recent open-heart surgery was already enough to explain her fear of death and panic. However the onset of severe reflux and oesophagitis made her recovery much more difficult, driving her to the brink of desperation.

As soon as she started getting proper treatment for her reflux, Mara felt much better. So she quickly began to emerge from the depression and panic, giving another clear example of how much suffering reflux can cause and how important it is to recognize it and treat it properly.

Giulia was a patient of mine who suffered from reflux from birth. It had "cleared up" by the time she was three or four years old. Then she came back to my surgery only for very occasional follow-up visits, until she was about 17 years old, when she began to suffer from depression and panic attacks. Her father, an excellent psychotherapist, turned to me in concern and with a little embarrassment: it seemed ironic that his own daughter, of all people, should be experiencing a serious emotional problem!

Giulia was a 22-year-old girl who was usually lively and interested in everything. She had changed, lost her sparkle and seemed downtrodden and subdued. She was a very clever singer and was training to become a professional performer. But recently her voice started failing her, deepening without any apparent reason. She was pale and tired because she could not sleep and had a perpetual stomach-ache and night-time cough. One day, while she was at school, she suddenly had her first panic attack. She felt as if she was losing control, her heart raced and she was scared she would die there on the spot, far from home, without her parents to comfort her. From then on, she began to live in fear that it would happen again. This fear was regularly confirmed, in a vicious circle that involved lack of sleep, stomach-ache and a choking sensation.

For me it was obvious that Giulia's condition was the result of a severe relapse of her original problem of reflux oesophagitis and prescribed the proper treatment for it. And (miracle!), she started soon feeling a lot better with her stomach and resting normally at night: the best psychotherapy she could get, which allowed her to recover a quality of life that she thought she had lost forever …

Barrett's oesophagus
If the reflux lasts for more than 20 years without proper treatment, the stomach acid can cause permanent damage to the oesophageal mucosa, which takes on an appearance described as *"Barrett's oesophagus"*. If this complication is suspected, the specialist takes small biopsies of the mucosa during oesophagoscopy to confirm the diagnosis.

A person with Barrett's oesophagus need not necessarily have more severe symptoms than other people. However, sufferers are more likely to experience symptoms that are more prolonged than other people and also some episodes of vomiting with blood. Barrett's oesophagus is much more common in men and people over 40. Although it does not cause any more suffering than a common case of oesophagitis, it is viewed with a certain amount of trepidation because it can be a precursor to developing cancer. However, this eventuality is always somewhat rare and can be foreseen and prevented.

ADULT DIAGNOSTIC QUESTIONNAIRE

As usual, for reflux to be suspected, **you must score at least 10 and enter at least two of the symptoms shown in bold and underlined**.

1. **Did you suffer from reflux symptoms as a child and/or adolescent?**
   For this purpose, complete the previous questionnaires.
   Yes................................5 points
   No................................0 points

2. **Do you suffer from stomach-ache, heartburn or spasms at the stomach entrance?**
   Sporadically....................0 points
   Often............................3 points
   Usually..........................5 points

3. **Do you have a sensation of bitterness and/or tastes coming back up into your mouth?**
   Sporadically................0 points
   Usually.......................5 points

4. **Do you have a lot of wind in your stomach and burp frequently?**
   Sporadically...............0 points
   Usually.......................3 points

5. **Do you have bad breath, especially in the morning?**
   Sporadically....................0 points
   Often............................5 points
   Usually..........................7 points

6. **Do you often hiccup?**
   Sporadically....................0 points
   Often............................3 points
   Usually..........................5 points

7. **Do you vomit from time to time without being apparently ill?**

Once a month……………...........2 points
More than once a month………..3 points

8. **Do you sometimes have considerable difficulty in swallowing solid foods?**
    No……………………………0 points
    Yes………………………...........3 points

9. **Do you experience spells when you become very pale and col lapse, almost as though you were about to faint**?
    No……………………………0 points
    Yes………………………...........5 points

10. **Do you have episodes of vomiting with blood**?
    No……………………………0 points
    Yes……………………………...5 points

11. Do you have a tickly cough only at night, without symptoms of a cold or other respiratory disorder?
    Sporadically…………….0 points
    Usually………...............3 points

12. Do you prefer not to eat breakfast because of an upset stomach?
    No……………………………0 points
    Usually…………….....................3 points

13. Are you constipated?
    Sporadically…………….0 points
    Usually………….............3 points

14. Do you get carsick or seasick?
    Once a year………..0 points
    2-3 times a year……..2 points
    whenever I travel…...3 points

15. Do you find it difficult to get to sleep after dinner?
    Sporadically................0 points
    Usually....................3 points

16. Do you wake up often at night?
    Rarely..................0 points
    Usually................3 points

17. Do you drink at night when you wake up?
    Rarely....................0 points
    Often.........................2 points
    Usually....................3 points

What if the problem is caused by Helicobacter?

In adults, infection caused by Helicobacter pylori is much more common than in children and adolescents and the possibility must always be excluded where there is a persistent stomach-ache. As time goes on, the effect can give rise to an ulcer of the stomach or duodenum. It can be mistaken for reflux because it causes the same type of pain and can be accompanied by episodes of vomiting, sometimes with blood. However, it must be remembered that whereas reflux is a very common problem, Helicobacter infection is much more unusual.

Helicobacter infection can generally be easily distinguished from reflux due to its characteristic symptoms.

1. It almost always starts in adulthood.

2. It does not occur with regurgitation and signs of oesophagitis: hiccupping, swallowing difficulty, vagal hyperstimulation spells and so on.

If in doubt, it is always best to carry out endoscopy of the oesophagus, stomach and duodenum for a definitive diagnosis. This examination shows inflammation in the stomach (which is almost never present with reflux) and the specialist can take small biopsies that reveal the presence of the bacterium directly when examined under the microscope.

TREATMENT OF REFLUX IN ADULTS

The principles of treating reflux in adults are the same as those discussed for adolescents. The more numerous and intense the symptoms, the more aggressive the treatment must be

Food and drinks

As usual, the foods *to be avoided are sweet things, particularly in the evening*. If possible, do not go to bed until at least an hour after finishing your evening meal. During dinner, limit fluid intake to the essential but drink water freely, although preferably in sips, for the rest of the day.

Alcohol

Drink alcohol with great moderation and avoid it altogether at the worst times.
Avoid chewing gum, which causes air to be swallowed and the uncomfortable phenomenon of a bloated stomach due to reflux.
Lastly, it is better to drink coffee only at breakfast time.

Avoid smoking

In addition to all the other damage it can cause, smoking impairs the function of the LES and this is another reason for avoiding it.

Sleeping position

It is noticeable that people who suffer from reflux instinctively try to go to sleep when they are in a sitting position. We all know adults who linger in the armchair after dinner, watching TV until the small hours, dozing and avoiding going to bed. By waiting longer before taking up a horizontal position during the early hours of night, their stomachs are already a little less full when they lie down and the reflux is less uncomfortable. If necessary, the most obvious way of avoiding a horizontal position when sleeping is to buy a motorized bed with a head that can be raised and lowered as desired.

Drugs

Adult reflux sufferers do not usually need constant drug treatment but *can limit themselves to taking medicines periodically whenever the disorder flares up.* When they become aware of the usual symptoms of heartburn, sensation of acid rising up into the mouth and so on, they should immediately start to take antacids and antisecretory agents **together**.

WARNING, this should NOT be done just as and when needed. It is much better to follow a proper course of treatment to be continued for at least two or three weeks, even you feel an improvement from the first day. Because the symptoms are due to oesophagitis, we cannot expect the inflammation to be cured after only a couple of days of treatment however quickly the symptoms die down.

I personally *prescribe lansoprazole, 30 mg in the morning* but you can use another antisecretory agent (omeprazole, pantoprazole, esomeprazole etc. at doses suggested by the specialist) and *an aluminium and magnesium hydroxide-based antacid, two chewable tablets or sachets 3/4 times daily. It is advisable to take the final dose of antacid at bedtime.*

Why should both drugs be given in combination and not one or the other alone? Because experience has taught me that using only one of the medicines is not enough to get rid of the oesophagitis.

After three or four weeks (the duration can be decided based on the rate at which the symptoms disappear) it is reasonable to stop treatment altogether and resume it if and when the condition flares up.

Remember the cases of Mara and Giulia? With episodes of *vagal hyperstimulation, oesophageal colic or vomiting with blood, I advise starting drug treatment at doses that are much more frequent than usual. During the first two days, for example, I prescribe a tablet (or sachet) of antacid every hour (even at night, if the pain causes waking) in addition to a dose of antisecretory agent in the morning.* In such cases, it is also advisable to continue the treatment for at least a couple of months, even though the symptoms seem gone earlier.

If relapses are frequent

If relapses recur more than two or three times a year and/or are particularly serious and/or esophagoscopy shows chronic damage (erosions, ulcers, Barrett's oesophagus), after initial treatment, it would be reasonable to establish *maintenance therapy. We could use an antisecretory agent given in alternate days in the morning, combined with a dose of antacid every day in the evening, before bedtime.*

What should be done during pregnancy?

If the burning sensation and spasms are very bad during pregnancy, it is absolutely fine for women to take aluminium and magnesium hydroxide-based antacids (Maalox, or Riopan), even at high doses, because these drugs are harmless to the foetus

Surgery

Surgery is advisable in the most serious cases, when any erosions and/or ulcers fail to heal (or recur continually), a large hiatus hernia is present, or Barrett's oesophagus is observed. This involves removing the section of impaired mucosa and/or carrying out the Nissen fundoplication procedure mentioned previously.

Laparoscopic surgery (keyhole surgery) is a much more established procedure in adults and ideal for achieving the intended purpose with as little discomfort as possible.

www.ingramcontent.com/pod-product-compliance
Lightning Source LLC
Chambersburg PA
CBHW072200170526
45158CB00004BB/1713